HERBAL
REVOLUTION

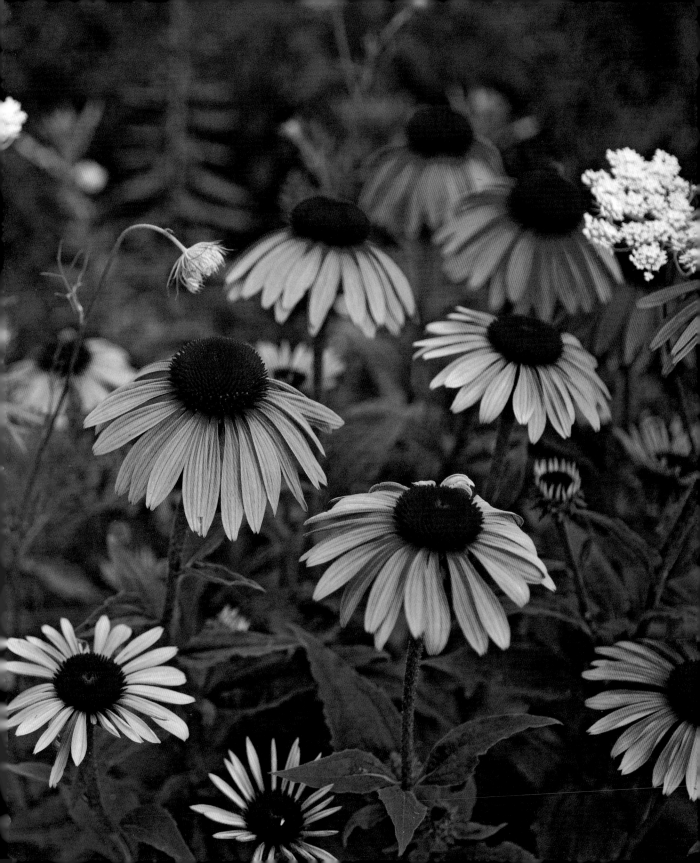

HERBAL REVOLUTION

65+ Recipes for Teas, Elixirs, Tinctures, Syrups,
Foods + Body Products That Heal

KATHI LANGELIER

Owner of Herbal Revolution Farm + Apothecary

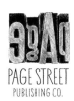

PAGE STREET
PUBLISHING CO.

PAGE STREET
PUBLISHING CO.

Distributed by Macmillan, sales in Canada by The Canadian Manda Group.

24 23 22 21 20   1 2 3 4 5

ISBN-13: 978-1-64567-050-6
ISBN-10: 1-64567-050-3

Library of Congress Control Number: 2019951603

Cover and book design by Ashley Tenn for Page Street Publishing Co.
Photography by Erin Little

Printed and bound in the United States of America

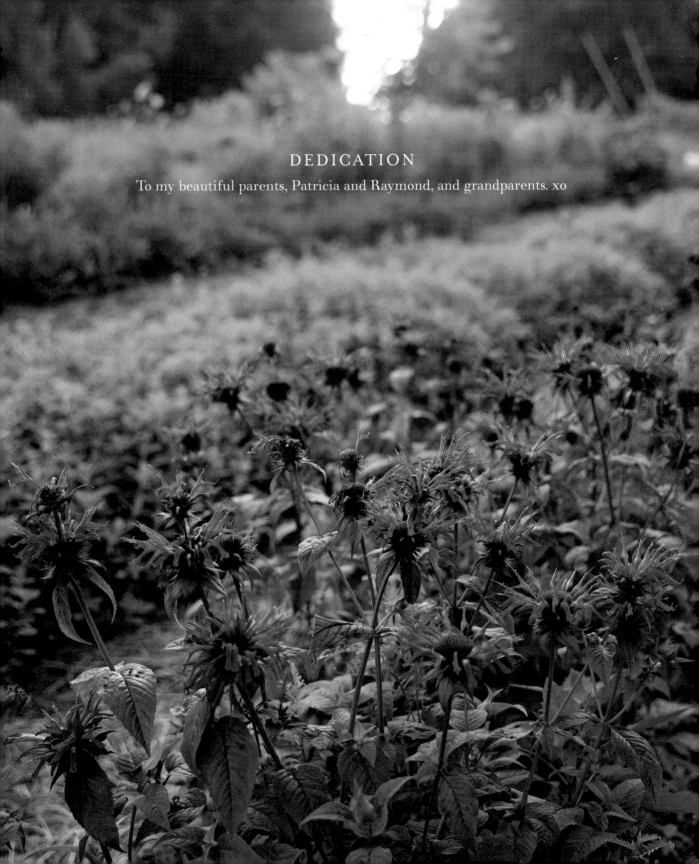

DEDICATION

To my beautiful parents, Patricia and Raymond, and grandparents. xo

CONTENTS

Keeping the Beat
Caring for the Physical + Emotional Heart 110

You Got This
Herbs to Support the Brain + Nervous System 130

Strength + Beauty from the Inside Out
Supporting Skin, Muscles + Bones 148

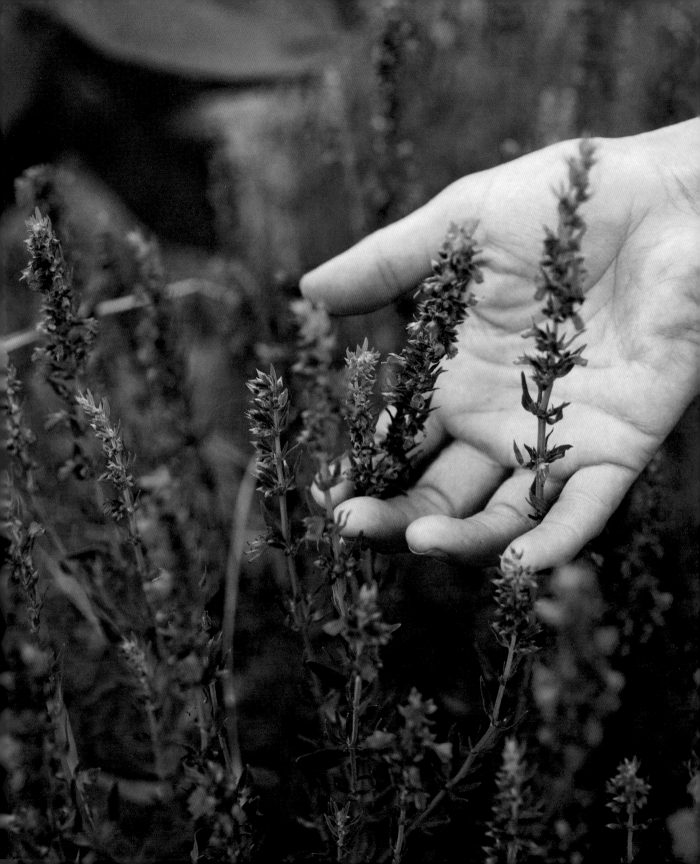

INTRODUCTION

I can feel the wind blowing on my face and bare arms as I walk to the upper growing field. I smile as I hear the sweet sounds of the wood thrush singing from the trees that run along the right side of the field. I approach the first plot and turn to walk through the tall hyssop aisles as I head to the chamomile patch in the plot beyond this one. The hyssop is in full bloom and their tall purple spires are buzzing and vibrating from the bumblebees and honeybees.

This daily action of walking outside in nature is an important one. These walks are meditative and open me to being in the moment. They provide me with information on how the plants are doing—are they happy, healthy and thriving? Or are they looking ill and needing some tending?

This practice helps me tap into my intuition and creativity. Medicine making for me has always been part intuition, along with critical thinking, science, historical evidence and a splash of creativity. If it weren't for my relationship with the plants, I wouldn't be making medicine or running an herbal business. I owe everything to them.

AN HERBAL BEGINNING

When I was six, my family moved from the city of Lewiston, Maine, to the farming community in Turner, Maine. I remember that feeling of wildness expanding. Suddenly, we went from having mostly houses surrounding us to a forest that nurtured my imagination, a place where I could run and play. I could disappear into another world, a world where the plants and animals talked with me.

I can't remember which memory happened first, but I do remember some of the first memories of tasting plants. They happened the first summer we moved into our new house. I'm guessing dandelion came first because it's first to bloom and I was obsessed with it, like most kids. I could rub it on my sister to make her skin turn yellow, and it had a thick white liquid that was sticky. I remember tasting that white liquid and how the bitterness seemed to run over every part of my tongue. It was intense, but I loved it even more. Red clover was next, this one being a very different experience. I remember picking each little flower and tasting the sweet nectar on the tips. The memory of that sweet nectar has stayed clear with me to this day.

I feel so fortunate to have grown up in rural Maine during a time when there were no computers or cell phones. I was able to spend most of my time outside, exploring the natural surroundings and learning the plants that grew around me, which ones I could eat and which ones were poisonous. In 1994, I moved to the coast of Maine, where I worked at a co-op and bought my first herbal books by Rosemary Gladstar and Deb Soule. I cherished these books and still do today. I pored over them by candlelight in my cabin and made every single recipe.

By 1995 I was teaching outdoor education, leading wilderness trips and apprenticing on farms. I went on to continue working on organic farms throughout my twenties in Maine, Vermont and California. Many of these farms grew not only produce but also medicinal plants. When they were putting up their food for the winter, they were also making their medicine. Between all the books I was reading, all the wilderness trips I was leading and the farms I was working on, my herbal foundations were growing.

By my early twenties I knew I wanted to farm, but it wasn't until around 2007, while in massage school, that I realized I wanted to grow mostly medicinal herbs, and not only that, but I wanted to start an herbal products business. I had been making my own herbal products for well over ten years, sharing them with friends and family, but then people started asking if they could buy things from me. I thought they were being nice. So in 2009, while attending my first herb conference, the International Herbal Symposium, I decided to enter the herbal products contest. I was looking to gain feedback on my formulas and blends from well-known experts in the field instead of just friends and family. To my surprise, I ended up winning first place in the categories I had entered, received great feedback and got to meet Rosemary Gladstar! It was such an uplifting experience to receive such powerful affirmation from an herbalist I had been looking up to for so many years. It truly gave me the confidence I needed to go home and create my company, Herbal Revolution.

AN HERBAL REVOLUTION

Herbal Revolution started as a passion, vision and dream, and I jumped in headfirst. Over the years, I've offered herbal tinctures, elixirs, vinegar tonics, teas, body products, herbal oils, flower essences, hydrosols, seed garlic and more. I started selling directly to my community through farmers' markets, events and fairs like the Common Ground Country Fair and through our website. Over the years we have grown and expanded to selling to co-ops, natural food stores and natural grocery stores.

To me, being a farmer goes far deeper than sowing a seed. On a daily basis, I care for the land, the insects and the animals. I'm a steward. I listen to the land every day. I'm a student of my surroundings and ecosystem, and a teacher of this knowledge about the food and medicine I grow. I believe sustainable farming can help support food security and health access to people in my community and throughout the country.

Herbal Revolution is now going into its tenth year. Holy, holy. We have a 23-acre (9.3-ha) farm with currently about 5 acres (2 ha) in medicinal herb and vegetable production growing for the Herbal Revolution products. I share the farm with my incredibly talented, handsome and ridiculously funny partner, Gus Johnson, along with a collection of goats, a donkey, a pony, chickens and cats.

About 2 miles (3.2 km) down the road from the farm in Union, Maine, is Herbal Revolution's headquarters. We have a production and manufacturing facility where the plants are dried and stored, and where all the products are manufactured and shipped out. The second building is in the process of being renovated into our retail store and café, where we will host events, music, herbal programs, classes and workshops year-round. We have so much exciting work going on, but it always comes back to the plants.

Herbal Revolution, the name, was inspired by dandelions and other plants bursting through sidewalks and up through concrete and pavement, saying, "F*** you! You can't hold us back." The resilience of these plants is beautiful, inspiring and motivating. If they can be this strong and resilient, then we can too. We can stand up to all the bullshit and make change happen, first within ourselves and then within our communities, which then will ripple out to other communities and continue from there. We hold a lot of power; it's easy for us to forget that.

Knowledge is power. The more knowledge you have about yourself, your body and ways to support your health through preventive care, the more power you have. I live in the United States, and this country's health care system is very good at tending to acute and emergency situations. It's truly amazing, and I couldn't be more grateful to the skilled doctors and surgeons who save lives every day. It's saved my life, my sister's life and my dad's life.

All that being said, I think the system is failing when it comes to preventive care, good nutrition and supplemental therapies. There is a lot of work that can be done to keep people from getting to full-blown heart disease, high blood pressure, diabetes and lung-related diseases caused by smoking.

This is where it's vital to educate yourself, understand your body and appreciate the risks that go along with eating certain foods, smoking, drinking, using drugs and living a high-stress life. This also means taking it a step further and understanding all the things you can do to support your body through foods, herbs and supplements. It can be so hard to change patterns. Many of these patterns can easily start as a way to cope with stress and trauma, but after a while those ways of coping become their own stressors on the body and add to your health risks. So the more you know, the more powerful you are!

SPREADING THE REVOLUTION

I felt moved to start an herbal business not just to make and sell products, but to create a life where I could talk about plants to others, to share the knowledge that I have learned and continue to learn. My goal has always been to help bridge the gap of food as medicine and medicine as food. Herbal Revolution is about creating opportunities to bring people and plants together. It's about empowering people to take control of supporting their health through the use of plants. It's about encouraging and inspiring others to take the step to starting their own herbal revolution.

I hope this book supports and nourishes you on your herbal journey and inspires you to become more connected with the plants. I hope it helps you become more curious, leaving you with eagerness to continue expanding your herbal knowledge and caretaking your body and health.

Thank you for being here with me. Thank you for wanting to work with the plants. And thank you for your support.

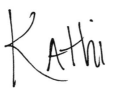

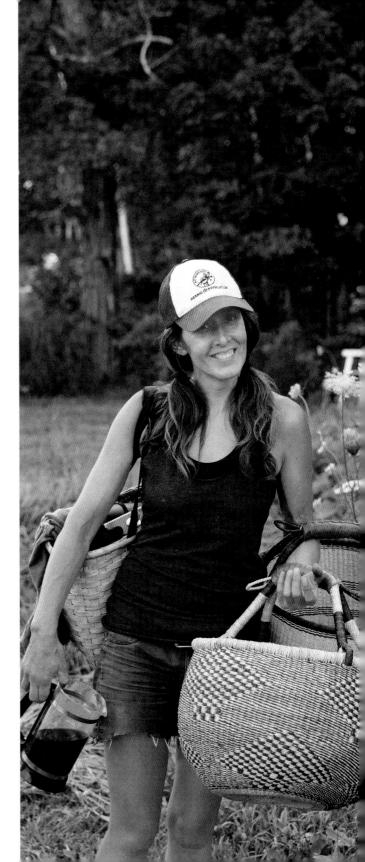

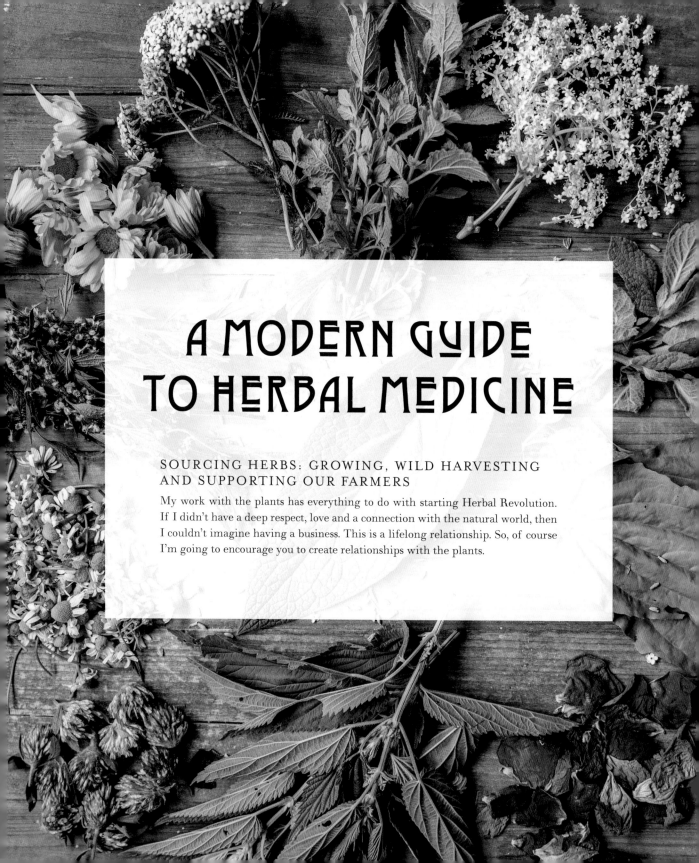

A MODERN GUIDE TO HERBAL MEDICINE

SOURCING HERBS: GROWING, WILD HARVESTING AND SUPPORTING OUR FARMERS

My work with the plants has everything to do with starting Herbal Revolution. If I didn't have a deep respect, love and a connection with the natural world, then I couldn't imagine having a business. This is a lifelong relationship. So, of course I'm going to encourage you to create relationships with the plants.

If you can, grow a garden with some herbs that are interesting to you, even if it's just a container garden in a window or on a porch. If you don't have either of those, then visit open garden spaces and botanical gardens, and take walks in the woods or down your street. Just walking down the street in a city I've found at least eight, but often way more, medicinal plants. These plants you wouldn't be able to harvest, but instead you can get to know them—how they grow, where they grow, whether they are resilient to heat and drought and whether they tolerate little sun and lots of rain. What do their leaves, stems and flowers look like? When do they flower? When do they go to seed? What do the seeds look like? All of these things play a role in learning more about each plant and how to work with it.

In the back of the book, you'll find some great seed and nursery companies I like to work with. So please, go and get dirty. Get your hands in the dirt and grow a relationship with some plants. In my opinion, this is where the medicine and healing begin.

You can also look for a local farm that grows herbs. A lot more farms these days are expanding from just growing produce, and more and more people are starting herb farms! Visit your local farmers' markets. While you're getting your veggies ask your farmer whether they grow any medicinal herbs or would consider it. Supporting your local sustainable farmers means you're supporting healthy farming practices, which grow healthy food, which provides you and your family with the best nourishment.

I always encourage either growing your own plants or purchasing from your local herb farmer, but if neither is an option, then there are some great herbal businesses you can order from online (see Resources, page 179).

For all your recipes, as best you can, I encourage you to use ingredients that are organic, non-GMO (screw you, Monsanto) and come from places that support sustainable practices. It can be done! Pretty much everything from what you put into your body and what you use topically on your body should be chemical free.

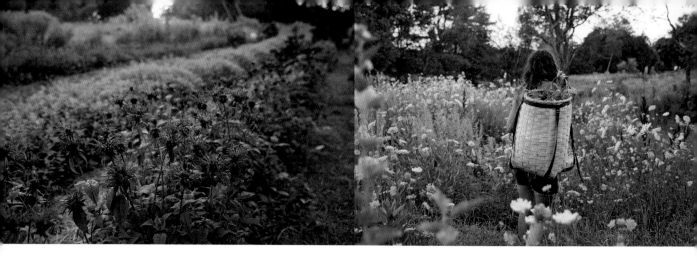

MY THOUGHTS ON WILD GATHERING

Throughout my life, I've traveled to the same special places time and time again to harvest certain herbs. When I did this, I would go through the checklist of what I was smelling (had the smell changed or was it the same?), what was I hearing (was it active in sound like the year before or not?) and what I was seeing (how did the stand of plants look; were they in abundance and healthy or was there less?).

There would be years I'd see less of one plant to the point that it should not be harvested. When this happened, I would sit and think on that plant. I would think about why I was harvesting it to begin with. I would meditate on the energy and medicine it offered. These moments I spend with the plants have been profoundly awakening and centering to my senses—especially the sense of listening to my gut and helping me tap into my intuitions and feelings. There are times when we absolutely need to use the plants internally or topically in order to receive their medicine, but there is also a great deal of medicine and lessons to be learned from just being with them, observing and paying attention to their habitat and listening to them.

Each year I would also see some plants in abundance. I would check in and explore whether there was a reason I might be seeing more of these plants. Was it because I needed to pay closer attention to it? Did it offer a medicine that I, my family or my community need more of? And so on.

Wild gathering is magic. It's how I first started working with plants and did for many years before I started growing so much of my own because there simply weren't any other places where I could get herbs. Over the years, I've come across many people who I feel shouldn't be wild gathering due to lack of knowledge and skill to safely and respectfully wild gather. This is one of the main reasons I hardly do it anymore, and I encourage people to grow their own instead. I only wild gather a few things these days, and only if the plants say it's okay. Last year, they said no.

Because this book is not focused on growing, harvesting and wild gathering, I'm going to strongly encourage you to hold off on wild gathering and stick to either growing your own or supporting an herb farmer. Wild gathering requires knowledge, skill and deep intuition. If you have this, great. But if you don't, then please wait until you've received more knowledge.

It's always of the utmost importance to ask for permission from the plants, but especially when wild gathering. You need to have a keen understanding of the plant's habitats, character, growth cycles and patterns. Most importantly, is it a plant of abundance, like dandelion or chickweed, or a plant that is rare, endangered or in threat of being endangered? Also, just because a plant is perceived to be in abundance doesn't mean it is. At this point, there are so many more herb farms growing plants that there is less of a need to wild gather. See the Resources section on page 179 for some recommendations.

A place to start is learning about the plants in your area that are endangered, threatened or at risk. You can find all this information at the United Plant Savers site (unitedplantsavers.org). I encourage you to become familiar with these plants so that you can avoid buying them if they are wild gathered and not farm grown.

LEARNING THE LINGO

As you expand your knowledge about herbs and herbalism, you will come across a few key terms, mainly *actions* and *energetics*.

ACTIONS

Actions describe the effects the plants have with the body. All herbs possess more than one action, so remember that plants are more than one thing, more than one action, and they work synergistically with other plants.

Having a good understanding of herbal actions will give you a much broader understanding of what the plants can do and how best to use them. It gives you more information so you can tailor your own recipes and formulas to your specific needs. Unfortunately, in this book we can't get deep into actions, but I do mention some of the actions the plants have in some recipes and in the section "The Plants" (page 168). There is also a brief glossary on the meanings of each action on page 178.

One particular action I do want to describe here is adaptogen. This herbal action is getting a lot of attention, and for good reason. Adaptogens are, for the most part, herbs that are tonic or nourishing. They are herbs that you can take on a regular basis to support the overall health and vitality of the body. Early work on adaptogens came out of the Soviet Union, and they discovered that these plants and mushrooms helped people adapt to environmental, physical and emotional stresses. Who doesn't need that? So you will see quite a few of the recipes in this book include herbs and mushrooms that are considered adaptogens.

To learn more about adaptogens, one of my teachers and mentors, David Winston, has a fabulous book called *Adaptogens: Herbs for Strength, Stamina, and Stress Relief.* This is a great book to have on hand in your herbal library. I refer to it regularly.

ENERGETICS

The energetics of herbs is another thing to learn about and consider when working with plants.

Energetics refers to how the plant literally works energetically within the body, as well as whether it's cooling, warming, hot, drying or moistening. Does it travel in an upward motion or does it travel downward?

I give a brief energetic profile on the plants in the section "The Plants" (page 168). Unfortunately, a deep exploration of energetics is outside the scope of this book, but I feel it's an important aspect to learning about plants, and I encourage you to read up on it. You can also take one of my herbal courses where we talk about it in depth.

HOW TO USE THIS BOOK

I realize you got this book so you could follow recipes, but if you're anything like me, you love to experiment and try different things. Learning about herbs isn't just about reading a recipe and following it. This is about your herbal revolution. Revolution and change don't happen from complacency; they happen when we use critical thinking. Question things and listen to yourself. What does your body want? What is your intuition telling you? What are the plants saying to you? The herbs we'll be working with in this book, just like me, don't like to stay within the lines of conformity. Plants by nature have order but are also incredibly rebellious. So, I encourage you to allow yourself the freedom to be creative, curious and rebellious, working with this book and beyond.

In this book, some of the recipes are written in parts. Writing recipes in parts is a method of formulating that is as old as time. It's an easy and simple way to work with plants because you can make as much or as little as you want. Parts can be any form of measurement you would like. You could use teaspoons, tablespoons, cups, ounces, etc.

Below is an example of how you could interpret parts in a recipe.

IN PARTS	IN TEASPOONS	IN TABLESPOONS	IN CUPS (WHAT I DO MOST OF THE TIME)
3 parts dried nettle	3 tsp dried nettle	3 tbsp dried nettle	3 cups dried nettle
2 parts dried milky oat tops	2 tsp dried milky oat tops	2 tbsp dried milky oat tops	2 cups dried milky oat tops
1 part dried raspberry leaf	1 tsp dried raspberry leaf	1 tbsp dried raspberry leaf	1 cup dried raspberry leaf

Most of the tea recipes in this book are written in parts, which makes it easy to mix up a big batch of tea blend to keep on hand, using cup measurements, or make a single cup using teaspoon measurements. Formulating recipes in parts gives you a lot of freedom to work with the plants and use what you have on hand.

HERBAL PREPARATIONS AND MEDICINE MAKING

There is something so magical, so radical and so humbling when it comes to making our own medicine. The work we do with the plants grounds us. It keeps us connected and tethered to our environment. Yet it also sends us into our subconscious and to the stars and back. Once we start to pay attention, we may notice that some of our dreams bring us lessons, answers or questions. Once you start working with the plants, you may notice that not unlike the ocean and the female body, the plants have cycles and rhythms that coincide with the moon. For many centuries, people harvested and made medicine in rhythm with the seasons on earth and the cycles of the sky. These practices are still carried out today by some, and there is a wonderful farming movement referred to as biodynamic farming. This type of farming embodies much more than the celestials, but planting and harvesting with the cycles of the seasons and the sky is a very important aspect.

Making medicine can also be a sterile, mechanical and scientific process. This isn't wrong. There is no wrong environment, as long as it's a safe space and you're clear and in tune with your intent.

As an owner of an herbal company, I have to follow a lot of regulations and procedures. So our processing facility is sterile and stainless steel and, at times, when you're wearing a white coat and a hairnet, it can feel like the magic is gone. But it isn't. The magic of medicine making lives within us, and has everything to do with our mind-set and relationship with the plants.

A great deal of the plants that we turn into medicine started as seeds on our farm. So I have seen those plants start from their beautiful seeds and spent the growing season tending to them before the harvest. Prior to having an herbal business, I would make the medicine right out in the fields, woods, coast, wherever. I still practice this method with my own personal medicine that isn't for the business. This is, of course, my preferred way of making medicine, but as I said, there is no wrong environment if your intent is solid.

So let's get to talking about the various ways to make medicine!

Tea: A tea is made by combining 1 cup (240 ml) of boiling water with 1 to 2 teaspoons of dried herbs or spices and letting it steep for 5 to 10 minutes. Typically, more fragile flowers, leaves and aromatic plants, which are high in volatile oils, make a wonderful tea. It is best to cover the cup to help retain those oils that may otherwise be lost in the rising steam. Some wonderful aromatics and flowers that make a lovely tea are mints, lemon balm, chamomile, lavender, bergamot, fennel, calendula and hibiscus. A typical dosage is 1 cup (240 ml).

Infusion: An infusion is a much stronger brew than a tea. Typically, an infusion will steep for 2 to 12 hours, or overnight, which allows more time to extract the medicinal properties from the plant into the water. An infusion is much darker in color and richer in flavor, creating a delicious and potent brew. Herbs that I love for infusions are nettles, oat straw, red clover and raspberry. All of these herbs create a deeply nourishing drink that is high in vitamins and minerals and can be enjoyed throughout the day.

To make an infusion, use 2 teaspoons to 1 ounce (28 g) (a large handful) of dried herbs to each 1 cup (240 ml) of boiling water, stir and then cover for 2 to 12 hours. I like to make my infusions right before bed. I take a 1-quart (960-ml) jar, place the herbs into it, pour the boiling water into the jar, stir the herbs, cover and let sit overnight. Come morning, it's ready to enjoy!

A typical dosage for an infusion is 2 to 4 cups (480 to 960 ml) daily for an adult, 1 to 2 cups (240 to 480 ml) for a child, and ¼ to ½ cup (60 to 120 ml) for a baby.

Decoction: A decoction is made with the roots, barks, seeds and berries of plants. It's a heated method and is the same process as making a reduction in cooking. When making a decoction, you're cooking the liquid down to at least half of where it started. So, if you started with 2 cups (480 ml) of liquid, you would simmer it to 1 cup (240 ml) or less.

I often like to start off first with an infusion, and then take that infusion with all the herbs, put it into a pot and reduce it from there.

To make a decoction, add 2 to 4 teaspoons (weight varies) of herbs to a stainless steel pot, pour in 2 to 4 cups (480 to 960 ml) of water and bring to a gentle simmer or to the point where it's just about to simmer. Keep it like this until the liquid has reduced by half, increasing or decreasing the heat as needed to maintain a gentle simmer.

The dosage is one-fourth the amount of what it is for an infusion. So, if the dose for an infusion is 1 cup (240 ml), the typical dose for the corresponding decoction would be ¼ cup (60 ml).

Syrup: Syrups are fun to make and taste delicious. Many traditional recipes use sugar, which helps make the syrup a thicker consistency; using raw honey or maple syrup (which I prefer) will make a syrup that isn't as thick. I prefer raw honey and maple syrup over sugar for a few reasons. One is the flavor. Another is that honey and maple syrup are locally produced where I live. Both have beneficial nutrients and vitamins, whereas sugar depletes the body.

When it comes to making syrups, I feel like almost any herb is up for grabs. Herbs that are very bitter, such as horehound, taste much better as a syrup than as a tea or an infusion. Often people make syrups with herbs that are soothing to the respiratory tract, but you can be creative and have fun with whatever herbs you choose.

To make a syrup, I use ½ to 1 ounce (14 to 28 g) of herbs per 1 cup (240 ml) of water. Sometimes I start off with an infusion, but ultimately, to make a syrup, you make a decoction. So if you started off with 2 cups (480 ml) of liquid you would reduce it to 1 cup (240 ml) or less. I tend to reduce mine even more than half.

Once the liquid has been reduced, you can then add the sweetener. Typically, syrups are made with a 1:2 ratio, such as 1 cup (240 ml) of decoction to 2 cups (480 ml) sweetener, which is intense and super sweet. Since we can store syrups in the fridge, it's no longer necessary to use so much sweetener as a preservative. So, you can easily do a 1:1 ratio and store the syrup in the fridge. A 1:1 ratio would be 1 part decoction to 1 part sweetener, or 1 cup (240 ml) of decoction to 1 cup (120 to 170 g) of sweetener. You can also add alcohol at the end to preserve it even further, using about 30 percent alcohol. You'll want to store in the fridge for up to 2 months. A typical dosage for syrup is ½ to 1 teaspoon up to 3 times a day.

Herbal Vinegar: We make a lot of vinegar tonics at Herbal Revolution. Certain herbs and vegetables combine brilliantly with cider vinegar. Raw apple cider vinegar alone is full of nutritional properties, such as vitamins, mineral salts and amino acids. When you combine cider vinegar with nutrient-dense herbs, the outcome is a food rich in antioxidants, vitamins and minerals.

Herbs easily release their minerals when infused in cider vinegar and make a wonderful addition to your food, such as in salads, sautéed greens and vegetables. Herbal vinegars are great for building bone density and addressing iron deficiency and are beneficial for those suffering from candida.

To make an herbal vinegar, fill a jar full with fresh-cut herbal leaves, stalks, flowers, fruits or roots that have been finely chopped. Then pour room-temperature cider vinegar into the jar until it is full. Cover with either a plastic lid or plastic wrap with a rubber band. You don't want to use metal, as it will corrode.

Label the jar with the name of the herb and the date that you made the vinegar. Place the jar in a cool, dark place and let the vinegar sit for at least 6 weeks. After 6 weeks, strain out the herbs and place in a beautiful glass container, label and enjoy!

Soup Stock: Stocks are another great way to use herbs and wild edible and medicinal mushrooms, which boost the immune system. Here in Maine, we have a lovely array of wild edible and medicinal mushrooms. The mushrooms you can buy at a store or order online include shiitake, maitake, chaga and reishi. They will add an earthy, hearty, meaty flavor to the stock. Some roots and herbs that go great in stocks are astragalus, burdock root, ginger, oat straw and nettles. Like all herbal preparations, let your imagination go and play around with different herbs for flavoring and nutritional benefits.

Tincture: A tincture is an extract often made using alcohol or a combination of alcohol and water. These solvents are also referred to as the menstruum, and the plant material is called the marc. We primarily use alcohol, because for most of the tinctures we make, the plants have alcohol- and water-soluble compounds, but some people use other solvents such as vinegar or glycerin. For the purpose of this book, the tincture recipes are made with 80 or 100 proof alcohol (see "A Note on Alcohol" on page 18).

At Herbal Revolution, we use 190 proof and dilute it with water to a certain percentage, depending on the solubility of the plant we're using. For instance, some plants need a higher percentage of alcohol, such as 85 percent, to extract certain compounds, whereas other plants may just need 35 percent. We are not going to get into all that in this book.

Here, we are using the folk method of medicine making. This is a method that has been used as long as alcohol has been around. It's where I started when I first made medicine. It's more of the eyeball method. So, instead of weighing a 1:5 ratio when using dried plants or 1:2 for fresh, I would eyeball and pack the jar I was using with freshly chopped plant material and then cover with the menstruum. I sometimes still use this method if I'm out in the field or woods making something for myself.

At Herbal Revolution, we primarily use the conversion method, but sometimes also the weight-to-volume method. The conversion method is most accurate and easy to replicate, which for an herbal businesses is incredibly important. To learn more about these various methods, check out *The Herbal Medicine-Maker's Handbook* by James Green.

Since this book is geared to working with plants year-round, all the tinctures are made using dried herbs, with the exception of milky oat tops. If you would like to use fresh herbs, I suggest using two to three times the amount that the recipe calls for to replace the dried herbs. If using dried herbs, you can grind them, if you have a grinder, or chop them, then place them in a jar and cover with alcohol. If using fresh herbs, you can either chop them by hand or run them through a blender and then place in a jar and cover with alcohol.

Make sure the alcohol is covering all the herbs and fills the jar. This may take a few times of shaking and stirring the alcohol with the herbs. Once you feel the herbs are fully covered and the alcohol is all the way to the top of the jar with no more air bubbles coming up, it's time to cap it. We let our tinctures sit for a minimum of 4 weeks, then strain and transfer to sterile bottles. During the weeks it's sitting, I recommend checking on the tincture, shaking it and tasting it. Clearly label the bottles with the date you bottled it, what it is, the plant's Latin name and the ratio.

The dosage depends on the plant being used and, of course, the person. But it's typical to use ½ to 1 teaspoon of tincture one to three times a day for addressing chronic issues using tonic herbs that are nourishing and for daily use. For acute issues, the dosage could be ¼ to ½ teaspoon taken every half hour, hour or couple of hours, until symptoms subside. Again, this is all very situational.

Herbal Infused Oil: There are, of course, a few different ways of making herbal oils, and I use different methods for different plants. For instance, I use the sun method with St. John's wort. I use freshly harvested blossoms, cover them in olive oil and let the jars sit out in the sun for at least 6 weeks. The sun method is important for St. John's wort, but other herbs, such as calendula, I dry thoroughly, then grind and then use a low heating method for 1 to 2 weeks or no heating method for 6 weeks. If I'm making an oil using roots, I tend to do either the low heat method for 1 to 2 weeks or the double boiler method for 4 hours. So it all depends. In this book, we are using the double boiler method because it's the quickest way to create an oil, but I encourage you to make the oils ahead of time and use the longer, slower process too.

If making it for myself, I usually eyeball the ratios, but again for the business we use the conversion method to get a consistent ratio of dried plant material to volume of oil.

Olive oil is the primary oil of choice for making an herbal oil. It's incredibly nourishing all on its own, but it's also the most shelf stable, which is very important. I also like to use sesame oil, which is heavy and warming and works well with warming roots and barks such as ginger and cinnamon. I often use sesame oil on joints and for hair. Coconut oil is another one I will use; it is lighter and more cooling on its own, so I like using it with cooling herbs, such as rose and peppermint. Rub infused oil into your skin as needed, starting with 1 teaspoon.

Salve: A salve is made by combining your infused oil with melted beeswax. The beeswax offers a layer of protection to the skin while also turning the herbal oil into a more solid form. How solid depends on the ratio of beeswax to oil used. Rub the salve into your skin as needed, starting with 1 teaspoon.

Lotions and Body Butters: These are all luscious ways of making topical herbal products. Lotions are the combination of both fats and water, where body butters are the combination of fats.

Lotions can be made using infusions, decoctions, floral waters, oils, butters and beeswax. There are limitless combinations. They have a much shorter shelf life and can easily mold, even with natural preservatives added. I tend to keep them in the fridge for this reason.

This book doesn't offer any lotion recipes, but you will find a body butter recipe in the Strength + Beauty from the Inside Out chapter (see page 148). Body butters typically are a blend of oils, butters and other fats and maybe some beeswax. Again, there are many combinations that you can come up with to create these. The ratios of each ingredient are the key to creating quality results.

And So Much More: Herbalists also make cordials, herbal beers, herbal wines, meads, drinking vinegars, smoking blends, honeys, herbal candy, lozenges, poultices, compresses, herbal baths, hydrosols, solid perfumes, suppositories, plasters, liniments, steams, washes, flower essences and beyond. This book is just the smallest scratch to the surface of working with herbs. If you are interested in expanding your repertoire, there are many excellent books and online resources to check out.

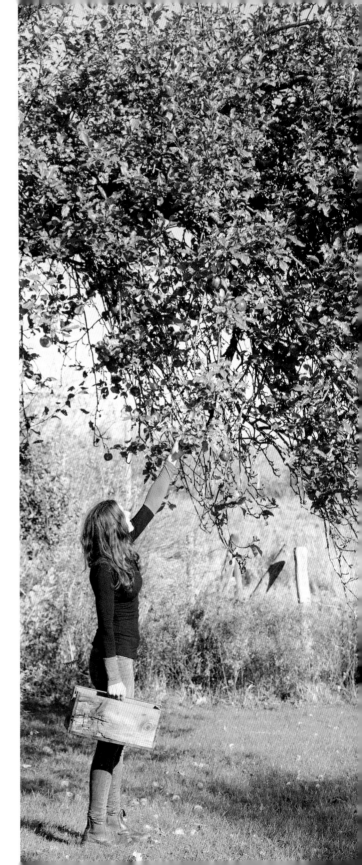

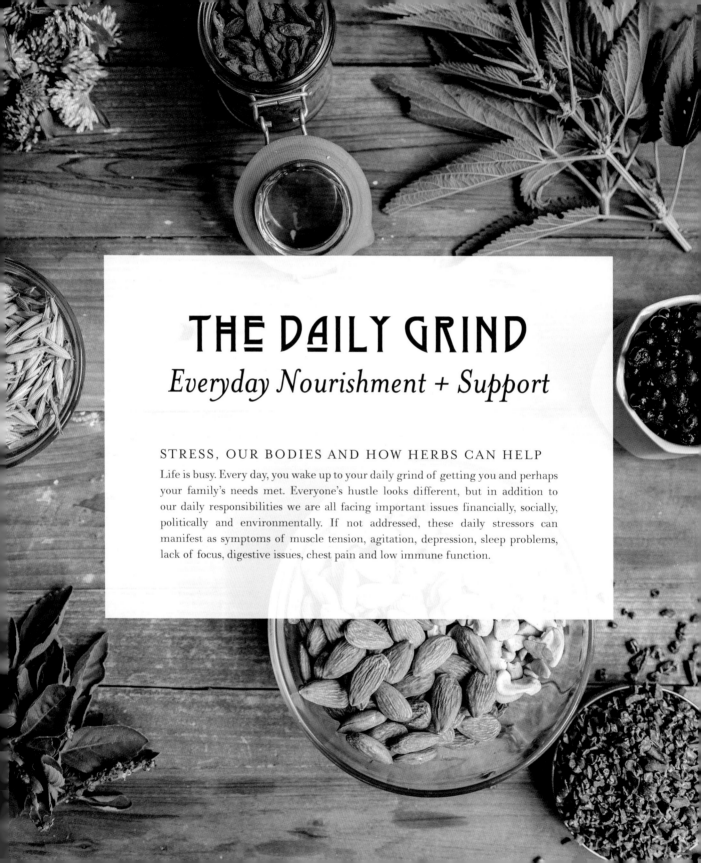

THE DAILY GRIND
Everyday Nourishment + Support

STRESS, OUR BODIES AND HOW HERBS CAN HELP

Life is busy. Every day, you wake up to your daily grind of getting you and perhaps your family's needs met. Everyone's hustle looks different, but in addition to our daily responsibilities we are all facing important issues financially, socially, politically and environmentally. If not addressed, these daily stressors can manifest as symptoms of muscle tension, agitation, depression, sleep problems, lack of focus, digestive issues, chest pain and low immune function.

The physical and emotional effect of stress on our bodies is real, and it is one of the leading causes of visits to the doctor's office. While we can't avoid stress completely, there are things we can do to support and nourish our bodies through the use of herbs, healthy foods, exercise, hydration and relaxation techniques such as yoga, qi gong and breathwork. The recipes in this chapter will help you make a little extra time to care for yourself.

When it comes to self-care and nourishment, I turn to the plants that are used both for food and for medicine, including nettles, kelp, dandelion, oats and mushrooms. These plants are often referred to as nourishing herbs, food herbs or tonic herbs. This is one of my favorite ways to work with plants. We all need to eat and drink, so working with plants within our daily routines of eating and drinking is a perfect way to access them.

In this section, I share with you some easy, basic ways to support and nourish the body as a whole. Many of these recipes are food recipes; some may even seem basic to you, and that's because they are. The goal isn't to overcomplicate or create recipes that require a lot of ingredients and time. The goal is to create easy, accessible and deeply nourishing recipes that you can fall back on.

USING ADAPTOGENS FOR STRESS

Adaptogenic herbs can have powerful effects when it comes to addressing stress within the body. I often roll my eyes at some of the trends I see in the health and wellness industry, but the use of adaptogens is one that I can get behind.

Adaptogens are a classification of herbs that have been proven to effectively strengthen our ability to deal with acute and chronic stress. To quote one of my teachers, David Winston, author of *Adaptogens: Herbs for Strength, Stamina, and Stress Relief*, "They help create a state of nonspecific resistance to stress (SNSR), they have little or no toxicity and have a normalizing effect on the body. They work by re-regulating the interconnected endocrine, immune and nervous system, as well as reproductive function, the enteric brain and our GI tract and cardiovascular function."

Adaptogens can help relieve symptoms of stress while also addressing the actual causes of the symptoms. Adaptogens are often referred to as tonic or nourishing herbs, which means they're herbs that can be used safely on a regular, daily basis. Some of my favorite adaptogens that you'll see featured in this chapter are ashwagandha, shatavari, reishi mushroom and tulsi, which you will learn more about in the following recipes.

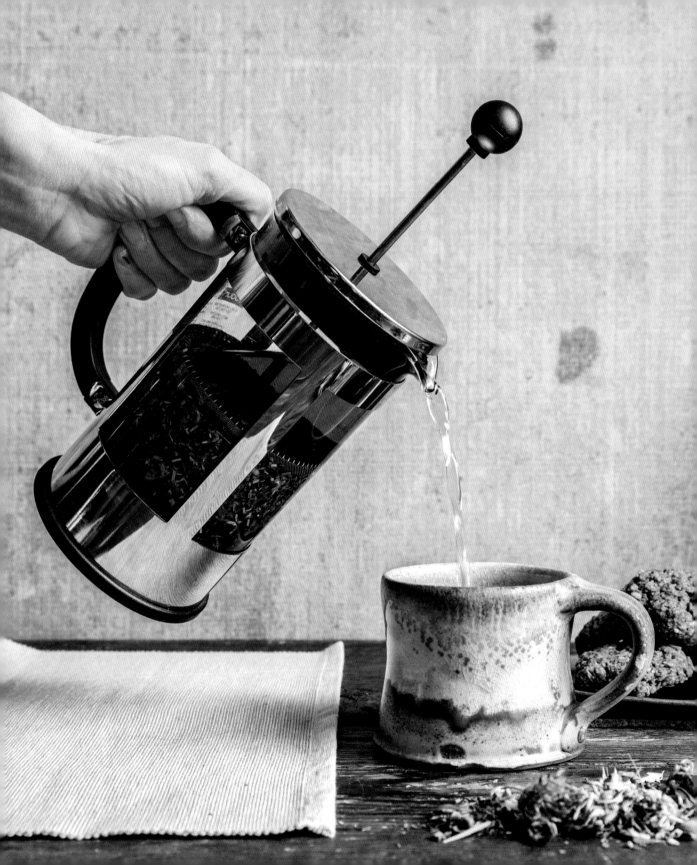

DAILY NOURISHMENT TEA + INFUSION

Yield varies

It's challenging to eat all the right foods and servings that our bodies need daily, especially in the off-season, when we have less access to fresh, vibrant vegetables, grown in healthy soil. Thank goodness for herbs! The great thing about herbs, especially nourishing herbs, is they can be used fresh or dried, year-round, and still be high in minerals and vitamins. The recipe below is a great blend of herbs full of minerals and nutrients, creating a nourishing, energizing and vital drink.

Some of the best herbs to use for infusions are nourishing herbs that are rich in minerals and vitamins, such as nettles, raspberry leaf, alfalfa and red clover. I also use tulsi, which is a fabulous adaptogen that is easy to grow and a wonderful herb to always have on hand for infusions, teas, syrups, tinctures and herbal honeys. I love using tulsi as a brain tonic for clarity. It helps clear out the fogginess and improve focus. It's a wonderful herb to take for anxiety and stress and uplifts the mood.

INGREDIENTS

2 parts dried nettle

2 parts dried milky oat tops

1 part dried lemon balm

½ part dried tulsi

½ part dried red clover blossom

WHAT YOU'LL NEED

Jar, for storage

Kettle

1-qt (1-L) jar or French press

Strainer

TO MAKE THE TEA BLEND

First, decide how much of the tea blend you'd like to make. I use cups for the parts, so I have a large batch that will last me a couple of weeks. When using cups, you will get about 6 cups (180 g) of the blend. If you're looking to make just a couple of cups of infusion or tea, then I suggest using tablespoon measurements, which will give you just under ½ cup (15 g) of blend.

Once you've figured out how much you want to make, start measuring the herbs into a mixing bowl. Get right in there and use your hands and mix the herbs until it all comes together into a lovely, cohesive blend. Store in a jar until ready to use.

TO MAKE THE TEA

Use a ratio of 1 to 2 tablespoons (3 to 5 g) of the herb blend to each 1 cup (240 ml) of boiling water. Place the herbs in a jar or French press and cover with boiling water. If using a jar, cover with a lid, and if using a French press, make sure not to press down on the herbs until after they've had time to infuse. Let it steep for 5 to 20 minutes, then strain into your favorite mug and enjoy warm.

TO MAKE THE INFUSION

Use the same ratio of tea blend to water as noted above. You can fill the French press or quart jar completely or just make a small amount, it's up to you. Once you've decided how much you'd like to make, place the herb blend into the French press or jar, and add the boiling water. If using a jar, cover with a lid, and if using a French press, make sure not to press down on the herbs until after they've had time to infuse. Let steep for at least 2 hours and up to 12 hours at room temperature. Strain and enjoy.

If you want to make a refreshing chilled drink, make the tea or infusion at night and place it in the fridge before bed. The next day, strain it and pour over ice and you have a delicious and refreshing iced tea infusion!

ROASTED ROOTS HERBAL COFFEE

Yield varies

Whether you can't drink coffee or you're looking to cut back, this is the perfect blend. Made with herbs that are earthy, bitter and rich in flavor, this blend can be supportive and building, where coffee for some can be depleting and taxing to the adrenals, liver and digestive system.

I like to use herbs such as burdock, dandelion and chicory, which are great for supporting the digestive system, including the liver. I also include astragalus root in blends to support the immune, respiratory and cardiovascular systems. Cacao is also wonderful for the cardiovascular system and is gently stimulating.

Because this isn't coffee, it can be enjoyed throughout the day without worry of afternoon jitters, anxiousness or insomnia, all of which can be caused by drinking coffee later in the day.

COFFEE

1 part dried roasted dandelion

1 part dried roasted chicory

½ part dried burdock root

¼ part dried maca powder

¼ part dried raw cacao powder and/or cacao nibs (optional, see Note)

⅛ part dried astragalus

OPTIONAL INGREDIENTS

⅛–¼ part dried ashwagandha

⅛–¼ part dried cinnamon chips

⅛–¼ part cardamom pods

⅛–¼ part dried ginger pieces

WHAT YOU'LL NEED

Jar, for storage

Kettle

Jar or French press

Strainer

TO MAKE THE COFFEE BLEND

First, decide how much of the coffee blend you'd like to make. I use cups for the parts, so I have a large batch that will last me a couple of weeks. When using cups, you will get about 3 cups (400 g) of the blend. If you're looking to make just a couple of cups of coffee, then I suggest using tablespoon measurements, which will give you around ¼ cup (36 g) of blend. For a single cup, use teaspoons.

Once you've figured out how much you want to make, start measuring the herbs into a mixing bowl. Get right in there and use your hands to mix the herbs until it all comes together into a lovely, cohesive blend. Store in a jar until ready to use.

TO MAKE THE COFFEE

Use 2 to 3 teaspoons (6 to 9 g) of coffee blend per 1 cup (240 ml) of boiling water. Place the herbs in a jar or French press and cover with boiling water. If using a jar, cover with a lid, and if using a French press, make sure not to press down on the herbs until after they've had time to infuse. Let it steep for 15 to 30 minutes, then strain into your favorite mug and enjoy warm.

For a chilled drink, let it steep at room temperature for at least 15 and up to 60 minutes before placing in the fridge to chill. If you'd like a more robust flavor, which I prefer, then no need to strain before chilling in the fridge.

Note: There is a small amount of naturally occurring caffeine in cacao, but the amount in this blend would not be noticeable to most people, and it adds such a lovely flavor. If you need this totally caffeine free, simply omit the cacao powder/nibs.

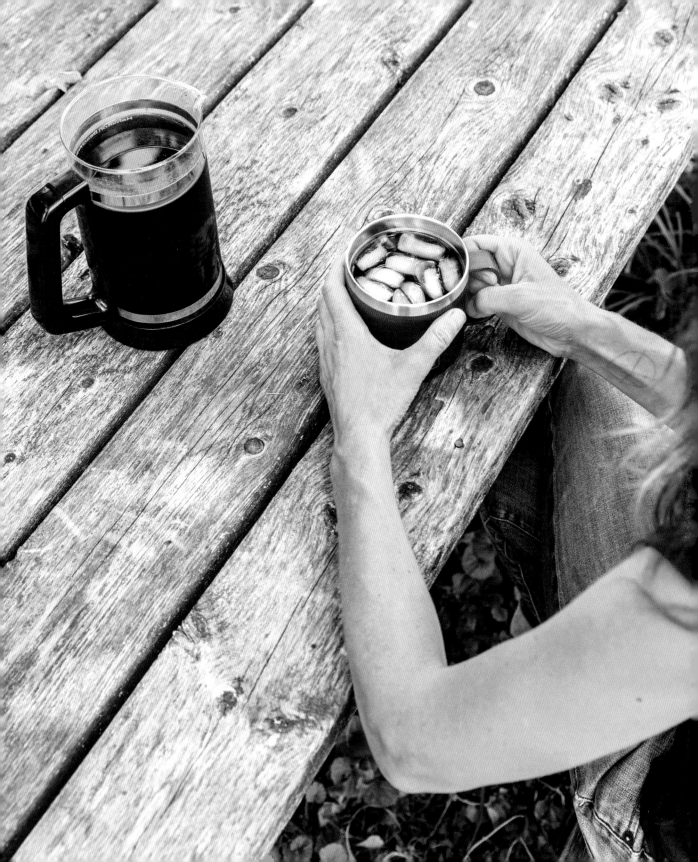

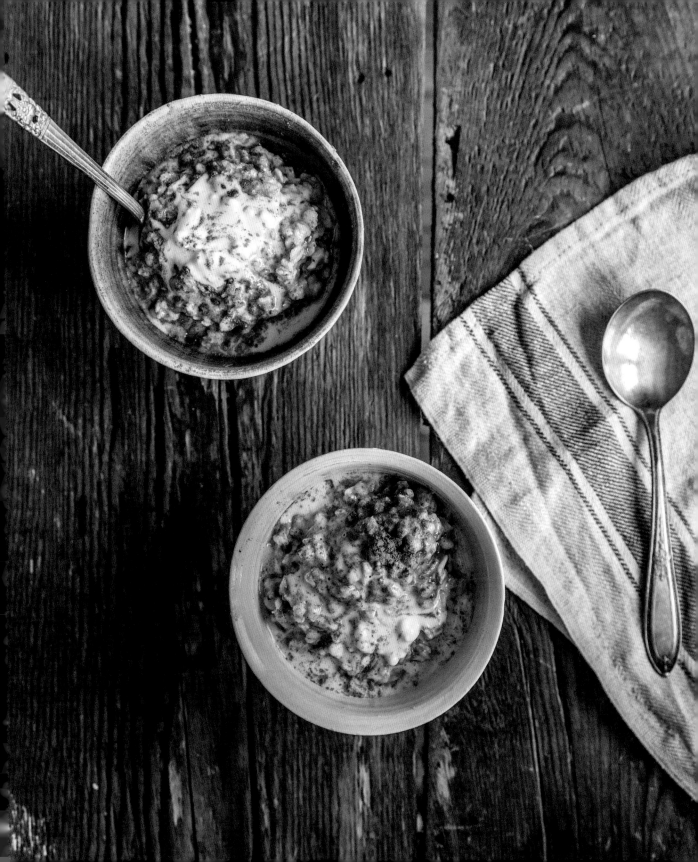

ASHWAGANDHA + CINNAMON OATMEAL WITH COCONUT CREAM + MAPLE SYRUP

Makes 2–4 servings

Oatmeal is one of my favorite comfort foods. It's so nourishing, and great for building and sustaining vitality, especially when paired with herbs and healthy fats such as coconut cream. Oats are a fabulous source of fiber, and when eaten regularly, they support the nervous system and the cardiovascular system, helping to control cholesterol, triglyceride and blood sugar levels.

Ashwagandha is a wonderful adaptogen that I especially like to use for nourishing the nervous system. I tend to combine ashwagandha with herbs and spices such as cinnamon. Along with being delicious, cinnamon is wonderful for the gut, circulation, the brain and increasing energy and vitality. Who doesn't need that!

INGREDIENTS

1 (13.5-oz [400-ml]) can coconut milk

4 tbsp (44 g) whole flax seeds

1 cup (118 g) rolled oats

½ tsp ashwagandha powder

2 cups (480 ml) water

1 tsp cinnamon powder

Maple syrup

WHAT YOU'LL NEED

Whisk

Spice grinder

Small pot

Open the can of coconut milk and scoop out the delicious, thick coconut cream from the top into a bowl, reserving the liquid.

Using a whisk, slowly add some of the liquid to the cream and whisk together until it becomes creamy and smooth. You can add more or less of the liquid depending on how thin or thick you want the coconut cream. It will thicken back up once it's put back in the fridge. Reserve the cream for the oatmeal, and drink the extra coconut liquid or place in the fridge for another use.

Using a spice grinder, grind the flax seeds into a meal. If you don't have a grinder, you can use preground flax meal. Add the oats, flax seeds, ashwagandha, 1 tablespoon (15 ml) of the coconut cream and the water to a small pot. Cook over low heat for 5 to 7 minutes or until the oatmeal reaches your desired consistency. Occasionally stir the oatmeal to keep it from sticking to the pot.

Serve in a lovely bowl and sprinkle cinnamon over the top. Pour additional coconut cream around the edge of the bowl and drizzle with maple syrup.

Note: This recipe is very adaptable. If you like your oatmeal creamier, use a higher portion of coconut cream and less water to cook the oats. Or you can use the plant-based milk of your choice instead of the water and coconut cream. Try different flavors and add-ins, such as dried fruits, nuts, other spices or other sweeteners like honey or an herbal syrup such as the Hawthorn Heart Syrup (page 126).

BLUEBERRY + CACAO SMOOTHIE WITH SHATAVARI

Makes 5–6 (8-oz [225-g]) servings

I'm always on the run in the morning, but I still want a healthy, nourishing breakfast. So, my go-to breakfast is this blueberry smoothie. It's filled with healthy fats, proteins, vitamins, fiber and, of course, herbs. Blueberries are a low-glycemic fruit high in flavonoids and antioxidants. Oats and flax seeds are great sources of fiber and vitamins and help thicken the smoothie. Spinach blends up well, making it a great way to get greens into the morning meal.

Some of my favorite smoothie herbs are shatavari, maca and cacao. Shatavari is a great adaptogen that I use to help with fatigue and anemia. Maca is delicious and great for supporting vitality, and cacao nibs give the smoothie a delicious crunch while adding healthy fats, fiber and protein. Other herbs that are a nice addition are ashwagandha for overall nourishment and support for the nervous system, triphala for supporting healthy bowel function, and nettles and alfalfa for support with anemia, energy and for their rich nutrients.

This recipe makes a big batch. I like to store it in the fridge so I can grab it quickly on busy mornings. If you prefer to make only a couple servings, you can easily cut the recipe in half or quarter.

SMOOTHIE

6 tbsp (65 g) flax seeds

1 cup (118 g) rolled oats

3½ cups (840 ml) water, divided

2 cups (310 g) frozen blueberries

1 cup (30 g) fresh spinach, washed

2 tbsp (30 g) almond butter (I prefer crunchy but smooth also works)

1 tbsp (10 g) maca powder

1 heaping tsp (4 g) shatavari powder

2 tsp (8 g) cacao nibs

OPTIONAL ADDITIONS

1 heaping tsp (4 g) triphala powder

½–1 tsp ashwagandha powder

½–1 tsp cinnamon powder

1 tsp raw cacao powder

½–1 tsp nettle powder

½–1 tsp alfalfa powder

WHAT YOU'LL NEED

Spice grinder

Small pot

Blender

Using a spice grinder, grind the flax seeds into a meal. If you don't have a grinder, you can use preground flax meal. Add the oats, flax seeds and 2 cups (480 ml) of the water to a small pot. Cook over low heat for 5 to 7 minutes or until the oatmeal reaches your desired consistency. Occasionally stir the oatmeal to keep it from sticking to the pot.

While the oatmeal is cooking, place the blueberries, spinach, almond butter, maca, shatavari, cacao nibs and remaining 1½ cups (360 ml) of water in a blender. Add any of the optional ingredients you'd like, too. Start on low speed and blend for a few seconds, working your way up to high. Blend on high speed for 30 seconds or so.

Once the oatmeal is done, use a spatula to scoop and pour the oatmeal into the blender. Again, start on a low speed and work your way up to a high speed. Blend until it's all nicely incorporated and smooth.

If it's too thick for you, slowly add more water until you achieve the consistency you like. If it's not thick enough, next time use less water or add more oatmeal. Although the oatmeal is hot, the frozen blueberries will take down the heat. For optimum digestion, enjoy at room temperature, but chilled works as well if you prefer.

You can store the smoothie in the fridge for 2 days.

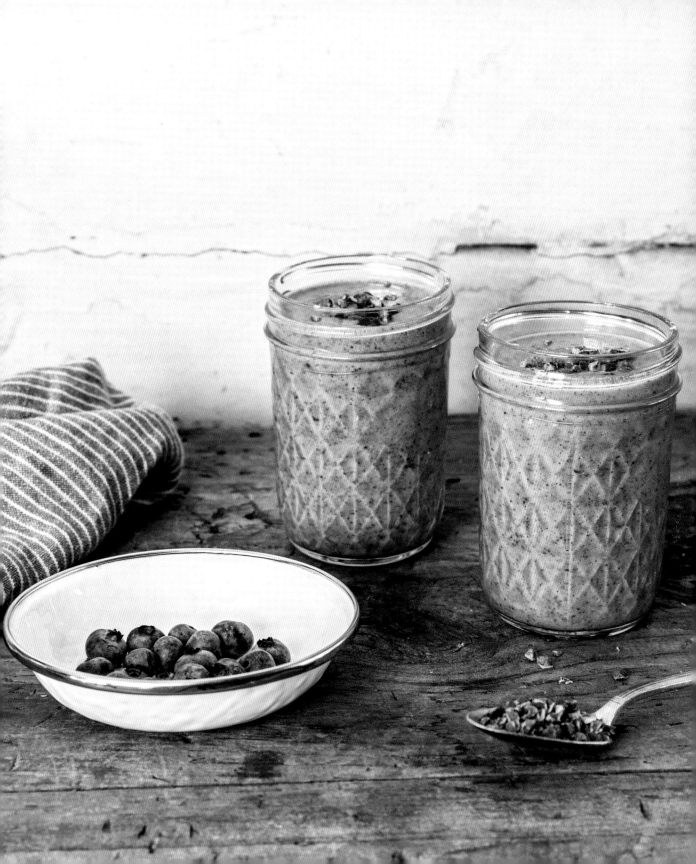

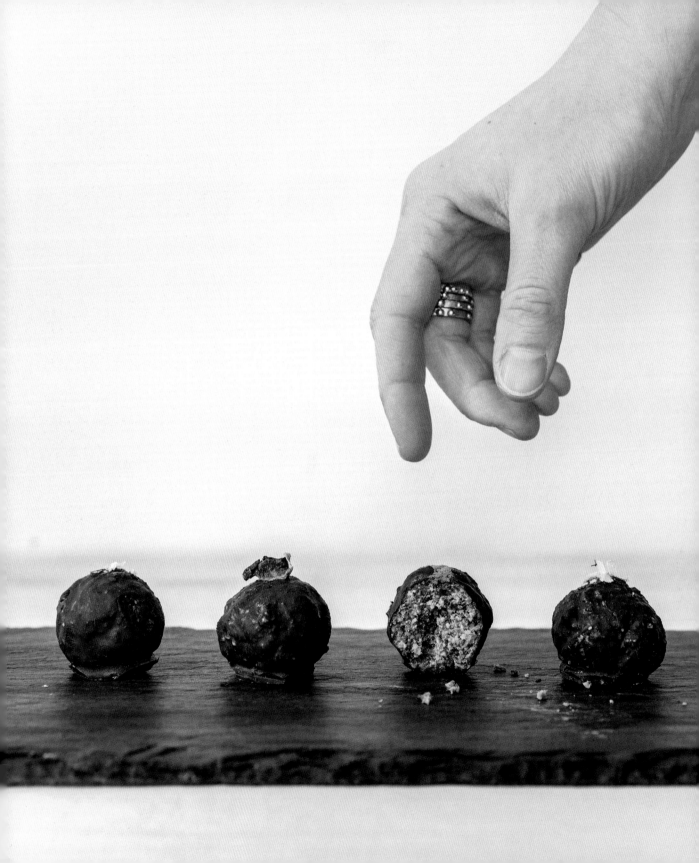

MACA + ASHWAGANDHA ENERGY BITES

Makes 6–8 small bites

Satisfying and filling snacks that pack a protein punch, like these tasty bites, are my favorites to have on hand. The cashews and almonds are a great source of protein, and coconut oil is a healthy fat that's nourishing to the nervous system. Dates offer a sweetness that's not only low glycemic but also nourishing to our bodies, especially in the colder months. Flax seeds are a great source of fiber, nutrients and omega-3 fatty acids.

I love ashwagandha: It's a fabulous adaptogen that we grow on the farm. It's a wonderful brain tonic that's nourishing to the entire nervous system. I use it to combat fatigue, brain fog, anxiety and sleep issues caused by stress. Maca is a delicious herb and has a traditional use for increasing energy, endurance and mood.

ENERGY BITES

1 tbsp (12 g) flax seeds

¼ cup (35 g) raw cashews

¼ cup (37 g) raw almonds

1 tsp maca powder

½ tsp ashwagandha powder

½ tsp cinnamon powder

Pinch of salt

2 pitted dates, at room temperature

½–1 tsp cacao nibs

¼ tsp vanilla extract

2 tsp (10 g) coconut oil, melted

CHOCOLATE SHELL

2 tbsp (30 g) coconut oil

2 tbsp (16 g) raw cacao powder

¼ tsp maple syrup or to taste

OPTIONAL TOPPINGS

Cinnamon powder

Flaky salt

Rose powder

Rose petals

WHAT YOU'LL NEED

Spice grinder

Food processor

Small baking sheet or plate

Parchment paper

Small saucepan

TO MAKE THE ENERGY BITES

With a spice grinder, grind the flax seeds to a meal. Alternatively you can use preground flax meal. In a food processor, combine the cashews, almonds, ground flax seeds, maca, ashwagandha, cinnamon and salt. Grind to a coarse meal. Add the dates and grind well. Add the cacao nibs and quickly pulse. Add the vanilla and melted coconut oil. Process until the mixture holds together. Remove the energy ball "dough" from the processor. Form into a ball and place it in the fridge for 15 to 30 minutes.

Line a baking sheet with parchment paper. Remove the dough from the fridge and roll into 6 to 8 small balls (about 1 teaspoon) and place on the prepared baking sheet or a plate. Place the balls in the freezer for 15 to 30 minutes.

TO MAKE THE CHOCOLATE SHELL

While the balls are in the freezer, make the chocolate shell. In a saucepan over low heat, warm the coconut oil until melted, then mix in the cacao powder. Add the maple syrup to taste. For a thicker shell, add more cacao powder and for a thinner shell use less. Once combined, remove from the heat.

Remove the bites from the freezer. Dip them in the chocolate and place back on the parchment paper or plate. Before the chocolate shell dries, sprinkle with cinnamon, flaky salt, rose powder, rose petals or anything else your heart desires, and place the bites back in the freezer for about 10 minutes. After they've chilled, you can get right to eating them or put them in a container and store in the fridge.

They keep for a week in the fridge, but I doubt they'll last that long. These bites go quick around here!

SESAME + NUT BARK WITH NETTLE

Makes 5–6 cups (300–360 g)

I love snacks that are healthy and functional and support the body's needs. Getting the right amount of proteins and nutrients such as iron and B vitamins is an everyday challenge. So, I try to consume a lot of foods and herbs that are rich in minerals and vitamins, such as nettles, raspberry leaf, alfalfa and kelp. This bar is made with a blend of seeds, nuts, herbs and natural sweeteners that are high in vitamins and minerals, especially iron and calcium.

I encourage you to play around with what your body is asking for. Maybe you want to go a more savory immune-supporting route and add some rosemary, thyme and dried garlic. Or maybe add some more nourishment with ashwagandha and cinnamon. For me, it's all about supporting my adrenals and consuming herbs that are rich in minerals and vitamins, so I make these with nettles, kelp and a pinch of sea salt.

I used to LOVE Cracker Jacks when I was a kid. I'd eat it with my mémère and pépère. Those days of eating foods like that are over, but this recipe totally hits the spot with the molasses and toasted nuts and seeds. So good!

INGREDIENTS

1 tbsp (6 g) powdered dried nettle leaf

1 cup (150 g) raw sesame seeds

¼ cup (36 g) shelled raw sunflower seeds

¼ cup (36 g) raw cashews, roughly chopped

2 tsp (8 g) kelp flakes

1 tbsp (20 g) molasses

¼ cup (60 ml) maple syrup

WHAT YOU'LL NEED

13" x 9" (33 x 23–cm) baking sheet

Parchment paper

Spice grinder

Preheat the oven to 350°F (180°C). Line a 13" x 9" (33 x 23–cm) baking sheet with parchment paper.

You can powder your nettle by placing some dried nettle leaf in a spice grinder and grinding until you have a powder. Measure out 1 tablespoon (6 g) of the powdered nettle and place it in a bowl. Add the sesame seeds, sunflower seeds, cashews and kelp to the bowl and mix thoroughly. Then add the molasses and maple syrup and mix everything until it comes together nicely.

Using a spatula or your hands, evenly spread the mixture onto the prepared baking sheet, covering the entire baking sheet.

Bake for 10 to 12 minutes. Your kitchen will smell delicious and nutty, and the bars should have a nice golden brown color around the edges and top.

Remove the pan from the oven and carefully place it in the fridge to cool for about 15 minutes. You can also leave it out to cool at room temperature; this will just take longer. Once cooled, break or cut into bite-size pieces. They should be nice and crunchy.

For a thicker, softer version, use a smaller baking sheet and spread the mixture out thicker. Cook for the same amount of time. Cool and break or cut into pieces. The bark shown in the photo is an example of the thicker version.

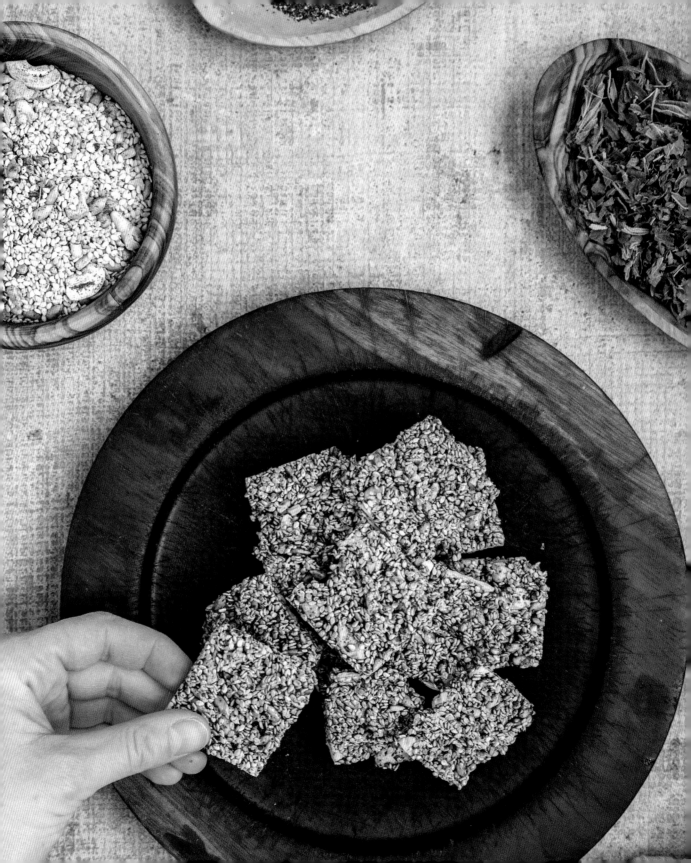

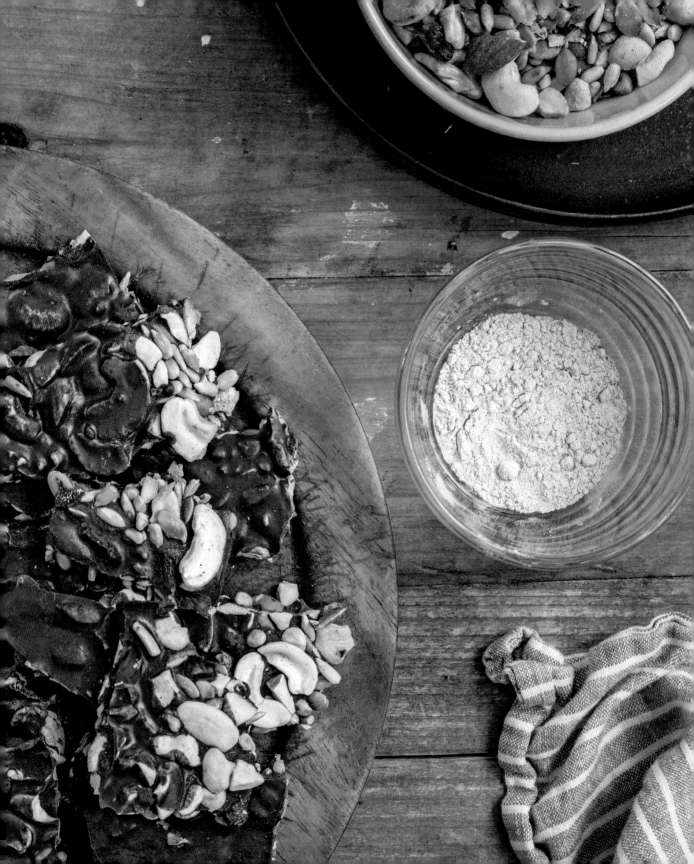

HERBAL CACAO BARK WITH ROASTED SEEDS + NUTS

Makes about 4 cups (440 g)

I love chocolate, but I don't love all the sugars often found in chocolate bars. I also love seeds and nuts. They're delicious and high in protein, healthy fats and antioxidants for supporting the body's daily nutrition needs. Cacao has a number of constituents that create the feel-good bliss we get when we eat or drink chocolate; it's also high in antioxidants and is a mild stimulant, a cardiotonic and an aphrodisiac. What more do we need!

These tasty bites are made with adaptogens—maca, eleuthero and ashwagandha—that are both nourishing and stimulating, making them a great midday snack when you need a healthy pick-me-up.

BARK

¾ cup (96 g) raw cashew pieces

½ cup (73 g) shelled raw sunflower seeds

¼ cup (40 g) raw almonds, chopped

3 tbsp (30 g) raw pumpkin seeds

1 tbsp (9 g) dried goji berries

Pinch of salt

⅓ cup (75 g) coconut oil

¾ cup (100 g) raw cacao powder

1½ tsp (6 g) maca powder

1 tsp eleuthero powder

½ tsp ashwagandha powder

1–2 tsp (5–10 ml) maple syrup

OPTIONAL ADDITIONS

¼ tsp cayenne powder

¼ tsp cinnamon powder

¼ tsp vanilla extract

WHAT YOU'LL NEED

Small saucepan

8" x 8" (20 x 20–cm) baking pan

Parchment paper

Set a small saucepan on low heat and, one ingredient at a time, dry-roast the seeds and nuts for 3 to 5 minutes. Be careful to not burn them; you want them to be roasted to a nice golden color. Place all the roasted seeds and nuts together in a mixing bowl. Add the goji berries and salt.

Next, using the same saucepan, add the coconut oil. The pan might be hot enough that you don't even need to turn the stove back on. Melt the oil and add in the cacao, maca, eleuthero and ashwagandha powders, mixing well. If it seems too thick, you can thin it out by adding a little more coconut oil. Once the powders are all smoothly incorporated with the oil, add the maple syrup and any optional additions.

Line an 8" x 8" (20 x 20–cm) baking pan with parchment paper and place the nut and seed mixture in the pan, spreading it evenly on the bottom of the pan. Take your herbal chocolate mixture and evenly pour it over the nut and seed mixture.

Place the pan in the freezer for about 20 minutes. Check to see if it's hardened. If not, leave it in for another 10 minutes and check again.

Once the chocolate is hardened, pull the parchment paper out of the pan and either break the bark into pieces or cut into bites. Store in a container in the fridge for up to 3 weeks.

NETTLE, ROASTED CAULIFLOWER + LEEK SOUP

Makes 8 cups (2 L)

Nettles are a true superfood. They are fabulous for supporting the adrenals and kidneys, and they're rich in protein, chlorophyll, vitamin C, fiber, silica, iron and so much more! Here on the farm, we harvest and use it fresh and dry it for tea and vinegar blends. Because it's loaded with minerals and vitamins, it's best to either eat nettles or make it into infusions, soup stocks and vinegars. If fresh nettles aren't in season or available in your area, you could try making this with baby spinach, but it won't have the same medicinal benefits.

I use maitake mushroom every time I make a soup stock or have time to set a pot on the woodstove and simmer it into a tea or syrup or make a tincture. Maitake supports immune health and function. This soup is an all-time favorite of mine. It's super easy, delicious and incredibly nutritious—the perfect way to awaken the body from its wintery slumber.

STOCK

3 cups (300 g) roughly chopped leek tops

1–2 whole carrots

1–2 celery ribs and/or handful of tops

3 qt (3 L) water

¼ cup (9 g) dried maitake mushrooms (pieces or powder)

Pinch of salt and pepper

SOUP

4 cups (400 g) sliced leeks (about 3 medium leeks)

1 large head cauliflower, roughly cut (about 8 cups [800 g])

Olive oil

Salt and freshly cracked pepper, to taste

8 cups (2 L) water

8+ cups (344 g) fresh stinging nettles

1–2 celery ribs, chopped

OPTIONAL TOPPINGS

Garlic olive oil

Grated Parmesan cheese

Fresh chive flowers

WHAT YOU'LL NEED

2 (3-qt [3-L]) pots

Strainer

2 baking sheets

Blender

TO MAKE THE STOCK

Roughly chop up all the vegetables, add them to a pot and add the 3 quarts (3 L) of water, mushrooms and salt and pepper. Bring to a simmer over medium-high heat, and then lower the heat to low and let it go for a few hours. I try to simmer for at least 2 hours, but depending on time you can let it cook longer. The goal is to have it reduce down to 4 to 5 cups (1 to 1.2 L). Once it's reduced, strain the stock and set aside.

TO MAKE THE SOUP

When the stock seems almost ready, preheat the oven to 400°F (200°C).

Place the leeks on one baking sheet and the cauliflower on the second one. Drizzle both baking sheets with olive oil, add a pinch of salt and cracked pepper and mix well. Place both baking sheets in the oven and roast for 20 minutes or until golden brown.

Meanwhile, in a 3-quart (3-L) pot, bring the 8 cups (2 L) of water to a boil. Using tongs, add the stinging nettles to the boiling water and boil for 2 to 3 minutes. Reserving the nettle water if you'd like (see Notes), strain the nettles and run them under cool water, then place the nettles in a blender. Add 1 cup (240 ml) of the soup stock to the blender and blend the nettles on medium-high speed until the mixture becomes a beautiful green puree.

Add the chopped celery to the blender and blend on medium-high for about a minute. Add the cooked leeks and cauliflower to the blender. Add 2 to 3 cups (480 to 720 ml) of soup stock and a pinch of salt, and blend on medium-high for 1 to 3 minutes or until you get a lovely puree. Continue to blend and add stock until you get to the consistency you desire.

Top with cracked pepper and any toppings of your choice.

Notes: Once the reserved nettle water is cool, I like to water my houseplants with it. You can do the same, or water your garden or find another creative use for the nutrient-rich water.

Be sure to take care and use gloves or tongs when working with fresh nettles to avoid touching the stinging leaves. Boiling removes the sting and makes them safe to eat.

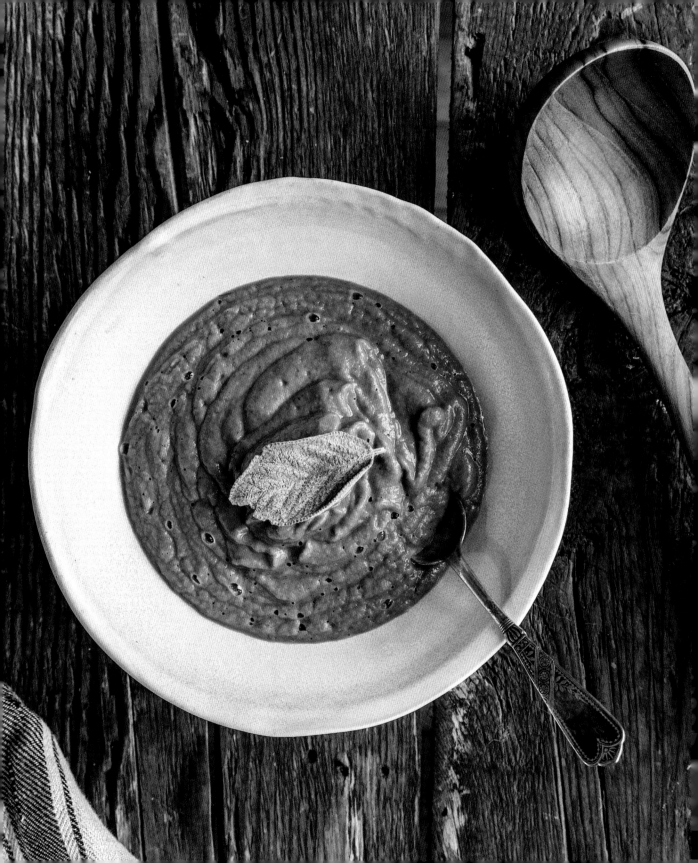

GO WITH YOUR GUT
Intuition, Creativity + Digestive Health

EVERYTHING IS CONNECTED

A great deal of my ideas for creating formulas happen while I'm out on the farm working with the plants. One day while harvesting in the beautiful chamomile patch, I was thinking about the medicinal benefits of chamomile and how everything is connected. The digestive system isn't just our stomach and intestines, it is also our mouth, esophagus, liver, gallbladder, spleen and colon, and still more. Much of the nervous system lives within the digestive tract, and research is starting to back up what many have intuitively known for years when it comes to the gut and mind connection. Hence the saying, "Go with your gut."

Because there are tons of nerves connecting the gut to our brains, what's happening in the gut shapes our emotions, mental clarity and creativity. Eating certain foods can leave our bodies feeling light and energetic, emotionally joyful and mentally clear, or they can cause us to feel heavy, weighted in our body, angry, frustrated, anxious, mentally blocked or foggy in the brain. When we think of the systems of the body, we often seem to separate them from one another, which sometimes is necessary when dealing with certain situations, but it's also important to remember that all the systems within our bodies are connected.

We intuitively feel and think from our centers; if the digestive system is off, then it can make trusting our guts more challenging. So, I believe it's important when formulating for the digestive system to always make sure to include nervines, which is easy to do. Many of our go-to digestive aromatic plants also support the nervous system. Plants such as chamomile, lemon balm, catnip and rose play a wonderful role in supporting all these areas.

DIGESTIVE FIRST AID

Our body gives us clear signs when our digestive system is not functioning at its optimum. Gas, bloating, belching, nausea, constipation and diarrhea are just a few common symptoms. Sometimes it's just something we ate and we can easily identify the issue, or these could be signs of something more chronic. When dealing with chronic issues, there may be other symptoms such as rashes, fatigue, pain and brain fog.

In this section, we have some go-to herbs such as chamomile, fennel and lemon balm that are great to call on when we're dealing with digestive distress. I recommend getting right to it and making these recipes, so you have them on hand when your gut starts to talk back.

If your gut issues are happening multiple times a week, every week, then you may be dealing with something more chronic. It can be helpful to step back and look at your eating and drinking habits and ask yourself some questions:

- What was your mood/stress level when eating?
- Do you sit down and eat, or do you eat on the go?
- How much water did you drink that day?
- What are the foods you're eating? Lots of red meat, dairy and processed foods, or whole grains, vegetables and fruits?
- Have you been on antibiotics recently or often?

One thing that you can do on your own is to try eliminating common food allergens. Sometimes it can be as simple as removing a certain food from your diet, and other times it can be far more complicated. The top foods I would suggest eliminating are wheat, eggs, dairy, nuts, nightshades, seafood, pork, corn, soy, sugar and anything containing gluten.

I realize the challenges that go along with an elimination meal plan. One way to ease into it is starting with foods that you already have a suspicion about. This way, you may be able to address the issue quickly. Other times, removing all these foods is the best way to start figuring out what's going on and whether it's food related.

When doing an elimination meal plan, it's best to remove foods for at least two to three weeks. After that time, then you'll want to slowly reintroduce foods back into your life, one at a time. It's important to give a few days in between the introductions so you have enough time to see how your body responds.

If you notice that your symptoms are more chronic, then I suggest you find a skilled practitioner, such as a naturopathic doctor, who can help assess your specific situation. I also recommend the book *Recipes for Repair* by Gail and Laura Piazza.

OUR LIVERS

Weighing in at over 3 pounds (1.4 kg), the liver is the second largest organ (after the skin) and the largest internal organ in our bodies. It's located mostly on the upper right-hand side of the abdomen underneath the lungs and diaphragm. It is triangular in shape and consists of two lobes, and its texture is solid and rubbery. The liver gets blood from two different sources, the digestive system and the heart.

The liver, also classified as a gland, performs over five hundred functions. So amazing! Some of these functions include processing nutrients, producing bile, detoxifying the blood, storing minerals and vitamins, and metabolizing fats and proteins. Oh, and the liver can regenerate! It can completely regenerate if there is up to 25 percent cell tissue left. It's the only organ that has this ability. Some of the major liver diseases are cirrhosis, hepatitis, fatty liver disease and alcoholic liver disease, which is the leading cause of cirrhosis.

There are many things that we can do to make sure our livers stay nice and healthy and filled with nutrient-rich blood. Start by eating foods that are balanced, stick to the important healthy fats and avoid processed foods, especially ones high in saturated fats. Keep alcohol consumption to a minimum, and the same goes for recreational drugs, as both can be incredibly taxing on the liver. It's important to give the liver plenty of support as well when dealing with diseases such as Lyme disease, and especially when taking antibiotics and other medications. Pharmaceutical medications can cause our livers to work overtime, especially if you're taking more than one.

It's important to include liver-loving herbs that can help support liver function and protect it. This includes turmeric, burdock root, dandelion root and artichoke leaf. These herbs are hepatoprotective, cleansing and bitter.

This chapter includes a mix of recipes featuring herbs that have a lengthy history of use for digestive, nervous and immune support—from your mouth to your colon. Enjoy the process of working with these plants as you tend to your body's needs. Listen to your body and how it responds to the plants; see what works and what doesn't work. I suggest adopting this practice with your foods as well. Now on to the recipes!

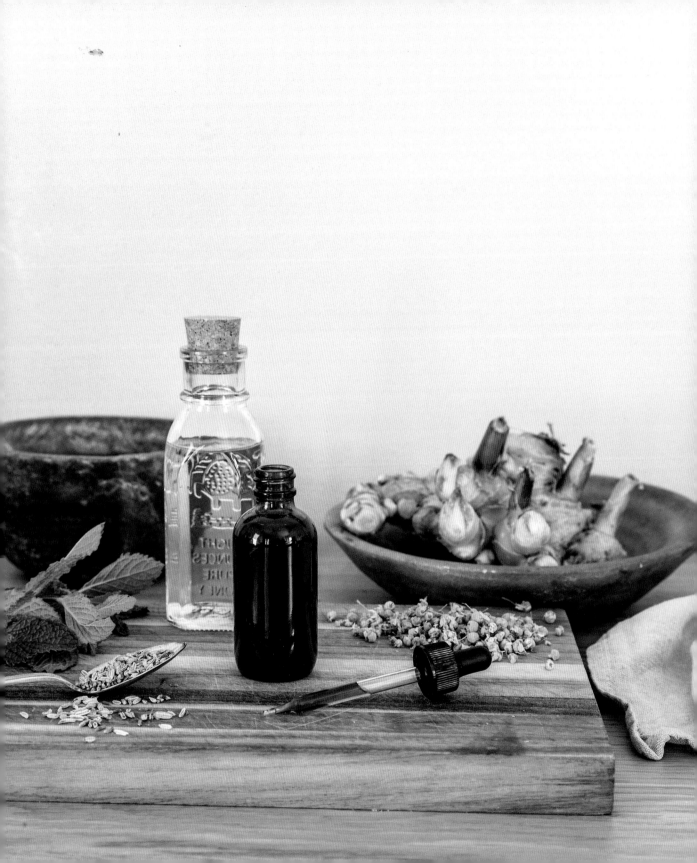

DIGESTIVE FIRST AID TINCTURE + TEA

Makes 6–8 oz (180–240 ml) tincture,
⅓ cup (22 g) loose-leaf tea blend

When my digestive system is feeling off and I'm looking for quick relief, I reach for aromatic plants, such as chamomile, fennel and peppermint. These are carminatives, which means they're great for relieving gas and bloating and for relaxing an upset and crampy digestive tract. Ginger brings warmth and circulation to this blend and is also a carminative.

This recipe can be made as either a tincture or a tea. I use both. I love the tincture for its accessibility and ease with travel. I also enjoy how making the tea asks us to be more mindful and slow down. If our stomach upset causes any anxiety or agitation, slowing down can be helpful in calming the whole system. I've also included a recipe for chamomile-infused honey. Raw honey is high in antioxidants and is a delicious way to work with aromatic herbs such as chamomile. It makes a wonderful sweetener for tea, syrups, tinctures and mocktails. I also enjoy a small spoonful now and again after my dinner as a sweet carminative treat.

CHAMOMILE HONEY (OPTIONAL)

2 tbsp (40 g) raw honey

2 tsp (2 g) dried chamomile

TINCTURE + TEA

4 tbsp (6 g) dried lemon balm

4 tsp (4 g) dried chamomile

1–2 tsp (3–6 g) dried ginger pieces

2 tsp (2 g) dried peppermint

1 tsp dried fennel seed

About 1 cup (240 ml) vodka

WHAT YOU'LL NEED

Small saucepan

Strainer

2 (8-oz [240-ml]) glass jars, one for the honey and one for the tincture or tea blend

Spice grinder

4 (2-oz [60-ml]) dropper bottles or a jar (for tincture)

TO MAKE THE CHAMOMILE HONEY

Place the honey and chamomile in a small saucepan and warm over low heat until the honey and chamomile are combined, 5 to 10 minutes. Turn off the heat and let it cool slightly. Repeat to gently infuse the honey without letting it come to a boil at any point. I usually repeat these steps a few times over the course of an hour or so.

You can either strain the chamomile out or leave it in and add it to your tea. If making for the tincture, I recommend straining the chamomile out. Store the honey in a glass jar in the fridge.

TO MAKE THE TINCTURE

Gather your herbs and one by one, measure them out and run them through your grinder, then place into an 8-ounce (240-ml) jar. If you don't have a grinder, you can just measure out the herbs and place directly in the jar.

Next, pour in the vodka until the jar is filled. Mix it all together and add more alcohol if needed, then place the cap on and shake. Open the jar back up and check to see if the alcohol level has dropped; if it has, add more to the jar and cover back up.

Label your jar and let sit for 4 weeks. Store in a place where you'll see it often. Shake it every week and taste a drop or two. After 4 weeks, strain into a bowl and add 1 to 2 tablespoons (20 to 40 g) of the chamomile honey if you'd like—so good. Bottle in labeled 2-ounce (60-ml) dropper bottles or a jar.

TO USE THE TINCTURE

Take 1 to 2 full droppers (¼ to ½ teaspoon) one to three times a day, straight or in a little water or tea as needed.

TO MAKE THE TEA

Measure all the herbs layer by layer into a small bowl, then thoroughly mix. Store in a glass jar. When ready to make the tea, use 1½ to 2 teaspoons (3 to 4 g) of the herb blend to 1 cup (240 ml) of boiling water. Let it steep for 10 minutes, then strain and enjoy with a spoonful or two of the chamomile honey if you'd like.

GUT-SOOTHING TEA

Yield varies

This tea blend is focused on soothing and repairing the intestinal tract. Years of eating inflammatory foods, taking medications such as antibiotics and living with stress can cause leaky gut syndrome, colitis, IBS, gastric ulcers, gastritis and other frustrating digestive issues to develop. This blend is made with herbs to help soothe and heal the lining of the intestinal tract and relieve painful spasms.

Calendula and marshmallow root are two herbs I reach for when it comes to soothing the digestive tract. Combined, these herbs are anti-inflammatory, gastroprotective, demulcent and soothing to inflamed mucous membranes, making this tea great for any digestive tract inflammations and irritations.

In this recipe, I've suggested some other herbal options that can be added if you're experiencing particular symptoms. This way, you can tailor it more to your needs.

TEA

2 parts dried marshmallow root

2 parts dried calendula

2 parts dried plantain leaf

1 part dried lemongrass

½ part cinnamon chips

¼ part dried licorice root

OPTIONAL ADDITIONS

For Gas and Nausea

2 parts dried fennel seed

For Gas Spasms

2 parts dried chamomile

For Diarrhea

4 parts dried yarrow

WHAT YOU'LL NEED

Jar, for storage

Kettle

Strainer

When making medicine, holding intent and vision is an important part of the process. As you're gathering your herbs, meditate on why you're making this tea blend, whether it's for yourself, a family member or a friend in need. Hold your reasons for making this medicine close to you while going through the following steps.

First, decide how much of the tea blend you'd like to make. I typically use cups for the parts so I have a large batch that will last me a few weeks or longer. If you'd like a smaller amount, use tablespoons, or use teaspoons for a single cup. Tablespoon measurements will give you about ½ cup (31 g) of tea blend. If using cups, you'll get about 7¾ cups (480 g) of tea blend.

Once you've chosen your measurements, gather the herbs and measure them layer by layer into a mixing bowl. Blend together with your hands and store in a jar.

To make a cup of tea, use 1½ to 2 teaspoons (1 to 3 g) of tea blend to 1 cup (240 ml) of boiling water. Steep for 10 to 30 minutes, then strain and enjoy.

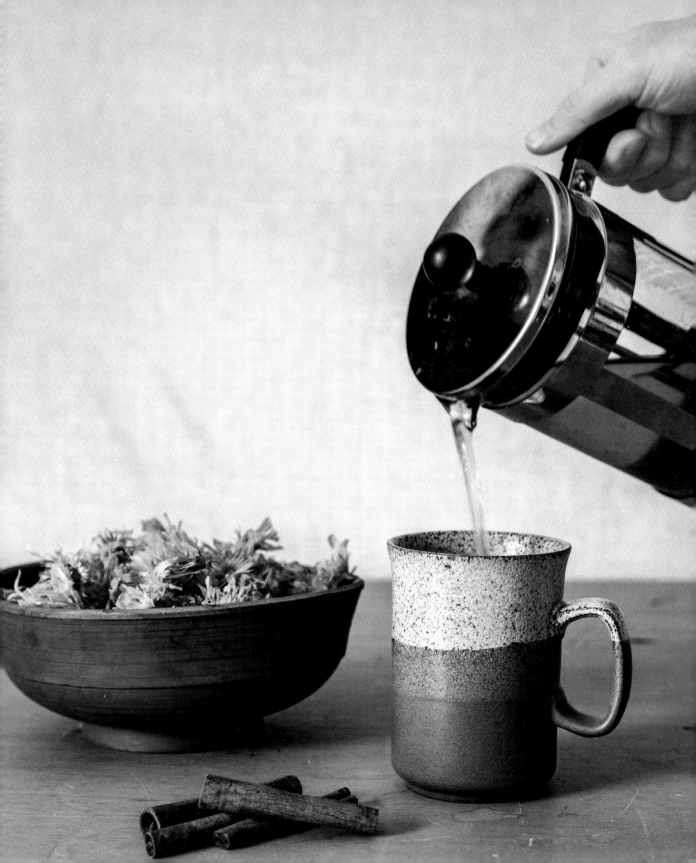

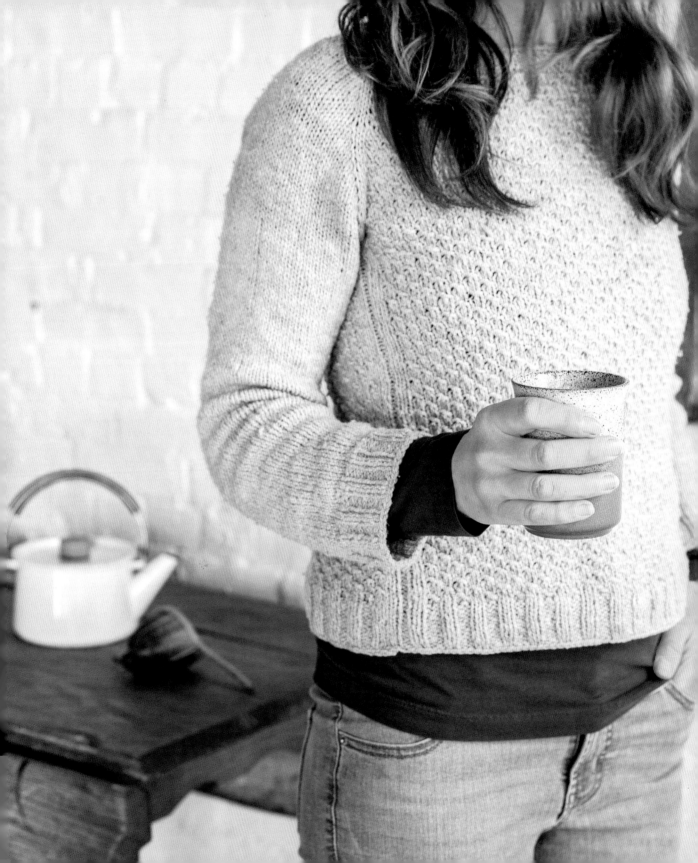

DAILY MOVER DECOCTION

Yield varies

Daily elimination is an important part of our daily health, clearing waste and toxins from our bodies. If we don't eliminate daily, we might start to feel fatigue, headaches and agitation. Herbs that I often turn to for supporting the digestive tract, healthy elimination and colon health are yellow dock, dandelion root and burdock root. Yellow dock is a wonderful bowel tonic and gentle laxative; it also supports liver function and bile secretion. Burdock and dandelion root are both great for supporting the growth of healthy gut flora, elimination and all-around digestive health. Combined, they make an earthy digestive blend.

Other everyday things you can do to help support daily elimination include drinking plenty of water, eating lots of healthy fiber, eating fresh fruits and greens, greens, greens, and making sure to include thoughtful movement in the day, such as exercise, dance, stretching or a walk.

Because this blend is made mostly with roots, the best way to prepare it is by making a decoction. You start with a certain amount of liquid and then simmer it down to a lesser amount, just like making a reduction when cooking. Roots, barks and berries work well as decoctions because they tend to be hard and woody. Simmering allows them more time to break down.

INGREDIENTS

2 parts dried dandelion root

2 parts dried burdock root

2 parts dried marshmallow root

1 part dried angelica root

1 part dried yellow dock root

1 part dried mint

¼ part dried licorice root

Honey, maple syrup or molasses, to taste (optional)

WHAT YOU'LL NEED

Jar, for storage

Small pot

Strainer

First, decide how much of the blend you'd like to make. I typically use cups for the parts so I have a large batch that will last me for a very long time. If you'd like a smaller amount, use tablespoons or teaspoons. Tablespoon measurements will give you a little over ½ cup (78 g) of tea blend; cup measurements will give you 9¼ cups (1.4 kg) of tea blend.

Once you've chosen your measurements, gather the herbs and measure them layer by layer into a mixing bowl. Mix the herbs thoroughly and then store in a jar.

When you're ready to make the decoction, use 2 to 4 teaspoons (6 to 12 g) of tea blend per 2 cups (480 ml) of water.

Place the herbs and water into the pot and place over high heat. Once the mixture reaches a simmer, turn the heat down and keep at a steady simmer until the liquid is reduced by half. Since we're starting with 2 cups (480 ml) of water, you want to simmer it down to 1 cup (240 ml), which takes 10 to 15 minutes. If you'd like to make a larger batch, simply keep the same ratios.

When ready, strain the decoction into a cup or glass. Feel free to lightly sweeten with honey, maple syrup or molasses. You can drink 1 cup (240 ml) all at once, or drink ½ cup (120 ml) and save the other half for tomorrow.

SLOW IT DOWN TEA

Yield varies

Just like constipation, diarrhea can happen occasionally because of something we ate or a stomach bug, or it could be a symptom of a chronic digestive issue. If you're dealing with diarrhea that lasts more than a few days, it's important to stay well hydrated and definitely try a cup or two of this tea. This tea blend is made with herbs such as raspberry leaf, cinnamon and lady's mantle, which are toning, astringent and supportive to the digestive tract.

Raspberry leaf is anti-inflammatory, antispasmodic, astringent and nutritive, making it a fabulous herb to help with mild to chronic diarrhea. Cinnamon is a carminative, so it can help relieve gas, bloating and cramps, and lady's mantle is a wonderful astringent herb that is effective for treating diarrhea. This is a great remedy to have on hand for occasional diarrhea and may also help with more chronic problems.

TEA

2 parts dried raspberry leaf

2 parts dried mallow

1 part dried nettle

½ part dried lady's mantle

¼ part cinnamon chips

OPTIONAL ADDITIONS

For Very Watery Diarrhea

½ part dried yarrow

For Cramping

½ part dried chamomile and/or fennel

WHAT YOU'LL NEED

Jar, for storage

Strainer

First, decide how much of the tea blend you'd like to make. I typically use cups for the parts so I have a large batch that will last me a few weeks or longer. If you'd like a smaller amount, use tablespoons or teaspoons. Tablespoon measurements will give you almost ¼ cup (8 g) of tea blend. Cup measurements will give you 5¾ cups (150 g) of tea blend. Once you've chosen your measurements, measure the herbs layer by layer into a bowl and mix thoroughly. Store the blend in a jar.

When you're ready to make the tea, use 1½ to 2 teaspoons (1 to 1.5 g) per 1 cup (240 ml) of boiling water. Steep for 10 minutes, then strain into your favorite mug and drink.

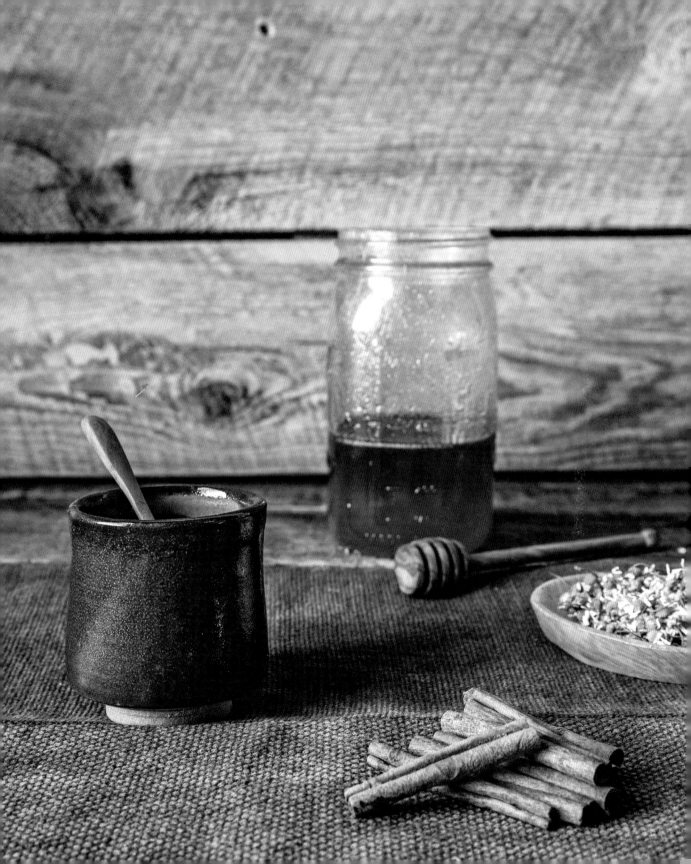

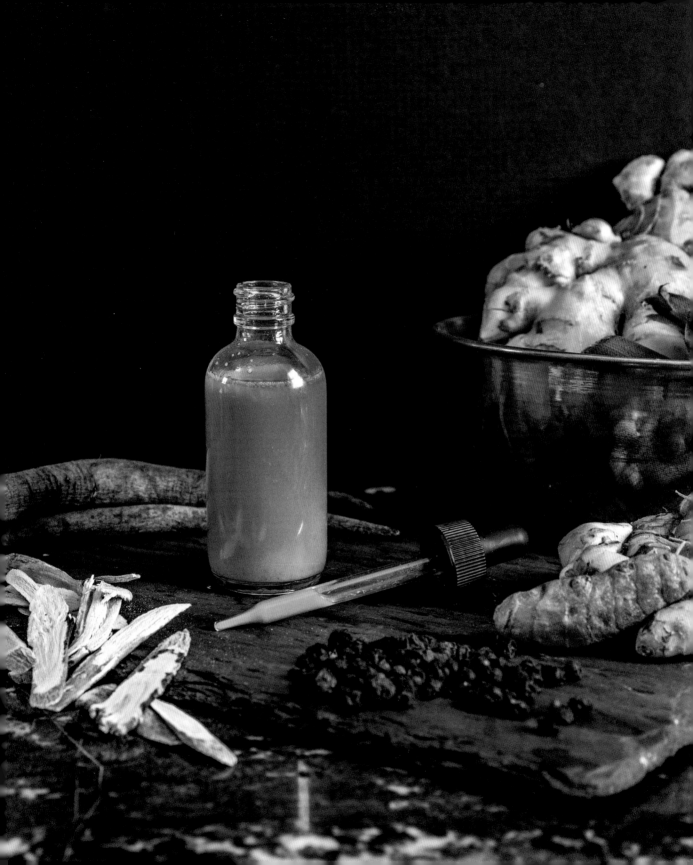

LOVE YOUR LIVER ELIXIR

Makes 6–8 oz (180–240 ml)

There are a lot of go-to herbs when it comes to supporting our livers, and one of my favorites is turmeric. Turmeric is high in antioxidants, has anti-inflammatory properties and is a hepatoprotectant, which means it specifically protects the liver! It also helps support the liver's detoxification functions.

I add turmeric to a lot of dishes and teas, but I also like having a tincture or an elixir on hand. I'm in love with this elixir. It's so tasty, and not only do I feel the benefits digestively, but I also feel the benefits in my joints. Tinctures are an easy and convenient way to access the benefits of turmeric. There are a lot of turmeric products on the market, and although there is some great research behind the standardized extract, I still prefer to use whole plant medicine. There are so many other constituents within turmeric that work synergistically with the well-known constituent curcumin. Black pepper and ginger both have this synergistic bond with turmeric, which is why it's best to combine at least one of them when making foods or herbal preparations with turmeric. In return, this will help our bodies more easily absorb and access the beneficial constituents.

INGREDIENTS

6 tbsp (54 g) finely grated fresh turmeric root

½ tsp dried ground black pepper

2 tsp (7 g) dried ginger pieces

1 tbsp (11 g) dried burdock root

1 tsp dried schisandra

1 tsp dried astragalus root

2 tbsp (40 g) honey (optional)

About 1 cup (240 ml) vodka

WHAT YOU'LL NEED

Microplane grater

8-oz (240-ml) jar

Spice grinder

Strainer

4 (2-oz [60-ml]) dropper bottles or a jar, for storage

Start by placing the grated turmeric root and ground black pepper into the 8-ounce (240-ml) jar. Gather the remaining herbs and one by one, measure them out and run them through a spice grinder, then place into the jar with the turmeric. If you don't have a grinder, you can just measure out the herbs and place directly in the jar.

Once all the herbs are in the jar, if using honey, you can add it now. Next, pour in the vodka until the jar is filled. Stir the herbs around in the jar and add more vodka if needed to top off the jar. Then place the cap on and shake. Open the jar back up and check to see if the alcohol level has dropped. If it has, add more to the jar and cover back up.

Label the jar and let sit for 4 weeks. Store in a place where you'll see it often. Shake it every week and taste a drop or two. After 4 weeks, you can strain and bottle into labeled 2-ounce (60-ml) dropper bottles or a jar.

TO USE
Take 1 to 2 full droppers (¼ to ½ teaspoon) before and after a meal, or as needed.

SPICED ORANGE BITTERS

Makes 6–8 oz (180–240 ml)

One of my herbal teachers, David Winston, often talks about how the average American is lacking in digestive acids and that most everyone should be using bitters in their daily routine, and I couldn't agree more. When we eat bitter herbs or take a bitter blend such as this one, it right away activates the digestive system, starting with our salivary glands. Our digestive juices start talking and waking up the system. This can help stimulate appetite, support the breakdown of food and encourage nutrient absorption.

I like to use bitter herbs such as orange peel, which is a fabulous tonic and carminative that helps enhance the digestion and absorption of foods. Artichoke leaf is another great herb that can help with sluggish liver and poor fat metabolism. It also can help stimulate digestion and absorption. I love burdock root and put it in most of my digestive formulas because it helps promote healthy gut flora in the digestive tract and it's also useful for liver stagnation.

One thing to keep in mind is that often a lot of bitter herbs are cooling to the body, so it's important to combine bitters with warming herbs. I like to use warming carminatives such as cinnamon and ginger to help keep the blend balanced.

INGREDIENTS

1 tbsp (11 g) dried dandelion root

1 tbsp (11 g) dried burdock root

1 tbsp (7 g) dried orange peel

2 tsp (8 g) cinnamon chips

2 tsp (6 g) dried ginger pieces

1 tsp dried cardamom pods

¼ tsp dried artichoke leaf

1–2 tbsp (20–40 g) honey (optional)

Vodka as needed to fill the jar

WHAT YOU'LL NEED

Spice grinder

8-oz (240-ml) jar

Strainer

4 (2-oz [60-ml]) dropper bottles or a jar, for storage

Gather your herbs and one by one, measure them out and run them through a spice grinder, then place into the 8-ounce (240-ml) jar. If you don't have a grinder, you can just measure out the herbs and place directly into the jar.

Once all the herbs are in the jar, if using honey, you can add it now. Next, pour in the vodka until the jar is filled. Mix it all together and add more vodka if needed to top off the jar. Then place the cap on and shake. Open the jar back up and check to see if the vodka level has dropped. If it has, then add more to the jar and cover back up.

Label your jar and let sit for 4 weeks. Store in a place where you'll see it often. Shake it every week and taste a drop or two. After 4 weeks, you can strain and bottle into labeled 2-ounce (60-ml) dropper bottles or a jar.

TO USE
Take 1 to 2 full droppers (¼ to ½ teaspoon) before meals. You can take it straight or in a small glass of water. It can also be used for making mocktails and cocktails that call for bitters.

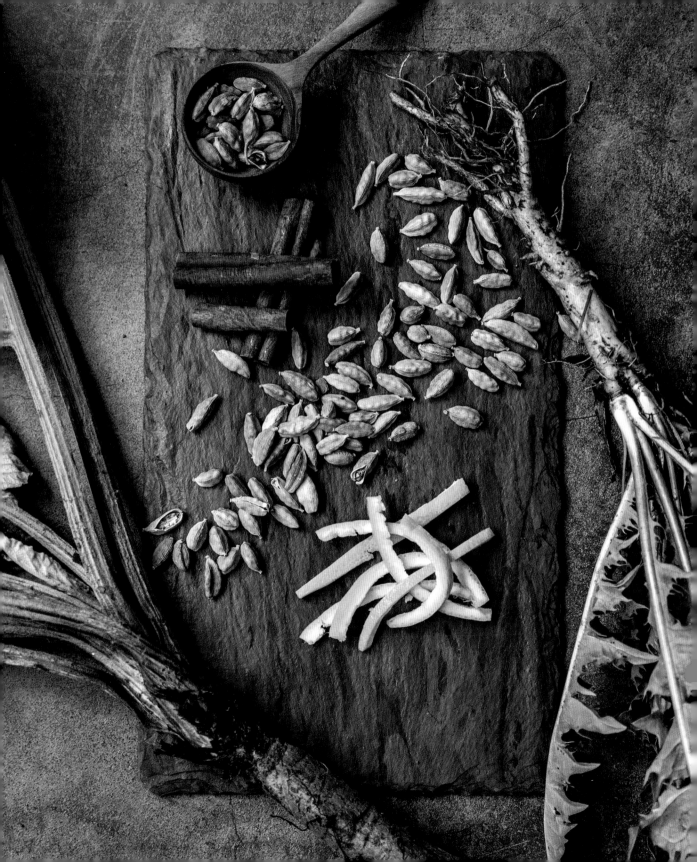

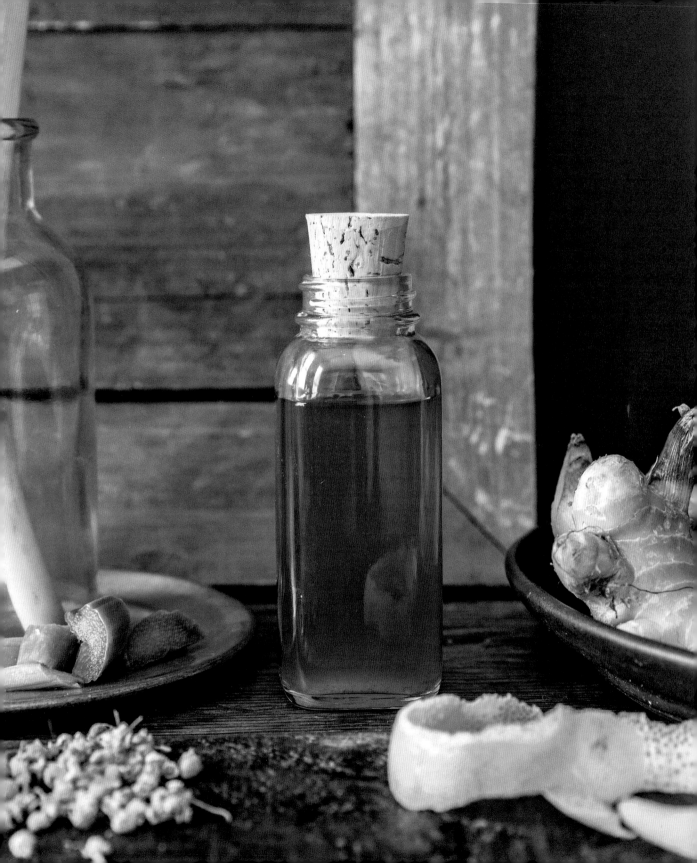

RHUBARB + LEMON DIGESTIVE BITTERS

Makes 6–8 oz (180–240 ml)

As an herbal farmer, I'm used to working with fresh plants, making medicine at specific times of the year. This is definitely a recipe that needs to be made either with fresh rhubarb while it's growing or with frozen rhubarb so you can make it year-round. I do both!

This is a lovely sour, tart bitter that is reminiscent of the summer. I really enjoy using this blend in the colder winter months when I'm needing to be reminded that the growing season is right around the corner. The sour and tart flavors of the rhubarb go great with the digestive-supporting lemon peel and lemongrass. I often like to use lemon peel in blends for its bitter energy and citrus flavor, and lemongrass is a wonderful digestive herb that is anti-inflammatory, not to mention delicious.

I've also listed some optional spices of fennel, anise hyssop and star anise; all three are wonderful carminatives and bring a lovely anise flavor to the blend.

BITTERS

¼ cup (36 g) diced fresh or frozen rhubarb stalks (see Notes)

1 tbsp (4 g) dried lemon peel (see Notes)

1½ tsp (5 g) dried ginger pieces

2 tsp (4 g) dried lemongrass

¼ tsp dried artichoke leaf

1 tsp dried chamomile

2–4 tbsp (40–80 g) honey (optional)

Vodka as needed to fill the jar

OPTIONAL ADDITIONS

¼ tsp dried fennel seeds

¼ tsp dried star anise

¼ tsp dried anise hyssop

WHAT YOU'LL NEED

8-oz (240-ml) jar

Spice grinder

Strainer

4 (2-oz [60-ml]) dropper bottles or a jar, for storage

Place the diced rhubarb and lemon peel into the 8-ounce (240-ml) jar. Then gather the herbs and one by one, measure them out and run them through a spice grinder, then place into the jar. If you don't have a grinder, you can just measure out the herbs and place directly into the jar.

Once all the herbs are in the jar, if using honey, you can add it now. If using any of the optional herbs, you can also add them now. I would choose only one of the three options unless you really like the flavor of licorice! Each of the optional herbs has a strong licorice flavor, so it may be overpowering to combine all three.

Add the vodka until the jar is filled. Mix it all together and add more vodka if needed to top off the jar. Then place the cap on and shake. Open the jar back up and check to see if the vodka level has dropped any. If it has, add more vodka to the jar and cover back up.

Label your jar and let sit for 4 weeks. Store in a place where you'll see it often. Shake it every week and taste a drop or two. After 4 weeks, you can strain and bottle into labeled 2-ounce (60-ml) dropper bottles or a jar.

TO USE

Take 1 to 2 full droppers (¼ to ½ teaspoon) before meals. You can take it straight or in a small glass of water. You can also use it to create mocktails and cocktails that call for bitters—oh yeah!

Notes: Make sure to purchase organic lemon peel as commercial lemons are highly sprayed.

Be careful to use only rhubarb stalks. Rhubarb leaves are toxic if ingested.

EAT YOUR WEEDS DANDELION + BURDOCK FRIES

Yield varies

The mascot and inspiration behind the name Herbal Revolution is the resilient dandelion, and our slogan is "Eat Your Weeds." In springtime, as the days start to become longer and winter starts to wane, I eagerly await the return of spring plants, many of which are bitter and fantastic for waking up the gut, especially if your digestive system is needing a boost after a sluggish winter.

Spring is a time of feasting. I love harvesting all the spring greens for salads, soups and sautés, but I also love the roots. Coming from the winter to the spring is still a chilly time here in Maine, so I like to slather dandelion and burdock roots with warming spices and roast them in the oven. So. Good. Roasting spring roots is the perfect way to transition our bodies from the dark, heavy months of winter to the lighter, brighter days of spring. This is definitely a recipe to turn to if you have access to fresh dandelion and burdock plants. I usually make a single serving with a handful each of burdock and dandelion roots, but feel free to make more if you have more roots available.

FRIES

Handful tender burdock roots

Handful tender dandelion roots

1 tbsp (15 ml) olive oil

Salt and black pepper, to taste

OPTIONAL SPICES
(A DASH OR TWO EACH)

Smoked paprika

Cayenne pepper

Smoked cayenne

Cumin

Nutritional yeast

WHAT YOU'LL NEED

Baking sheet

Preheat the oven to 350°F (180°C).

Thoroughly wash and dry the burdock and dandelion roots, making sure to cut off the green tops. Cut the roots lengthwise into the shape of thin fries. Place them on a baking sheet, drizzle with the olive oil and sprinkle with salt and black pepper. Then sprinkle on a dash or two of any or all of the wonderful spices from the options list. Mix thoroughly, making sure each fry gets nice and coated with oil and spices.

Place in the oven and roast for 10 minutes or until cooked to your liking. I like mine nice and crunchy, borderline burnt, so I usually leave them in a little longer for that texture. Just check on them every 2 to 3 minutes until they reach the desired roast.

These are so good and can be enjoyed with any sort of tasty aioli, hot sauce, vinegar or—my favorite—all on their own.

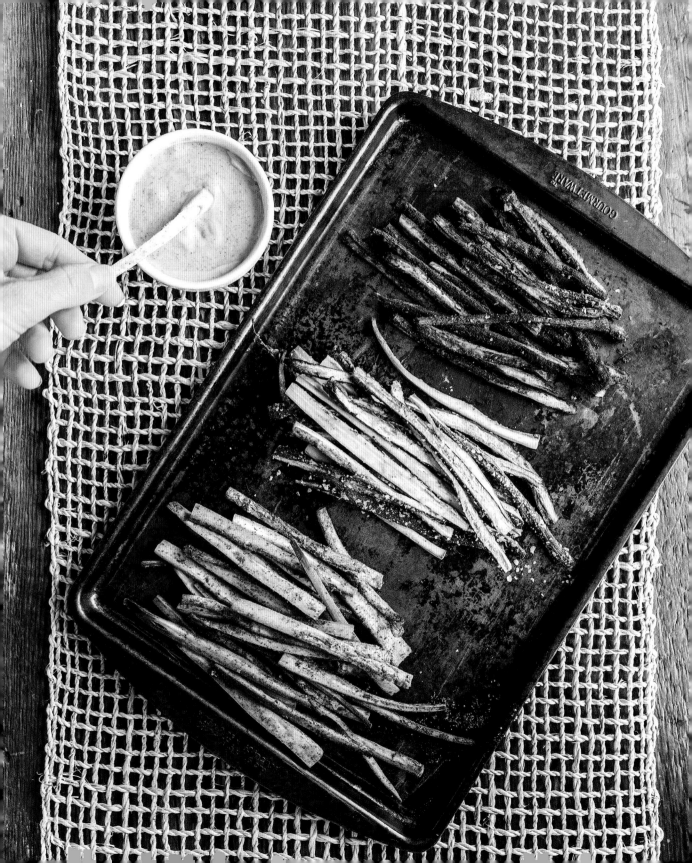

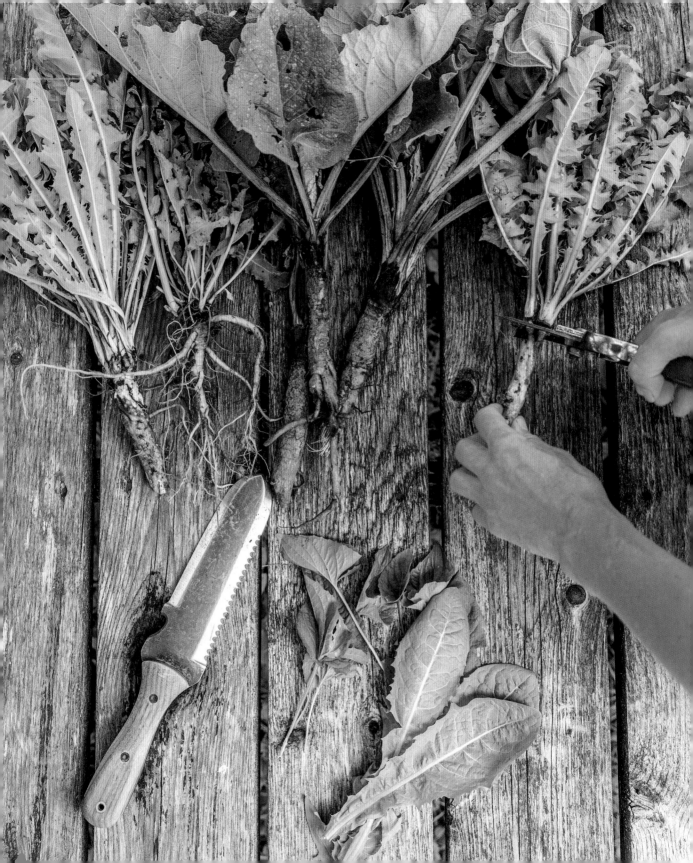

SPRING DIGESTIVE VINEGAR

Makes about 4 cups (960 ml)

Springtime is a brilliant time of year—with the return of light comes the return of plants. We start to shed the dark, heavy months of winter and sprout toward the sun, craving movement and lighter foods that are bitter (and therefore supportive to the digestive system) as well as mineral rich. Historically, spring is for eating nutrient-rich and bitter greens as they start to emerge from the ground. These plants are vibrant, brilliant and full of nutrients just waiting to be enjoyed! This vinegar is a wonderful way to harness the power of these nourishing plants while also supporting the digestive system.

I love using raw apple cider vinegar with herbs for many reasons, one being that it's a prebiotic food that most people have in their pantry. It's also a great solvent for extracting mineral-rich plants. Apple cider vinegar was one of the first methods of extracting herbal medicine dating back five thousand years! Because this is a spring tonic, it's best to make this using fresh plants, so if you don't live where these plants grow, connect with a local organic farmer or herbalist and they might be able to help you source these ingredients. If you can only find some of them, just use what you have.

As a reminder, if you plan to gather these plants yourself, be very careful that you are 100% sure on plant identity. If you're only 99.9% sure, then don't pick it! Also, make sure you pay attention to not harvest from places that may have exposure to pesticides, exhaust, road salts, etc.

VINEGAR

1 cup (68 g) fresh chickweed leaves and stems

½ cup (68 g) fresh dandelion roots

½ cup (34 g) fresh dandelion leaves

½ cup (68 g) fresh burdock root

½ cup (34 g) fresh violet leaves

¼ cup (34 g) fresh yellow dock root

2 tbsp (12 g) grated fresh ginger

Honey, to taste (optional)

Raw organic apple cider vinegar as needed to fill the jar

OPTIONAL ADDITIONS

Handful fresh or dried chamomile

1–2 tbsp (6–12 g) fresh or dried lemon peel

1–2 tbsp (7–14 g) fennel seed

1–2 tbsp (11–22 g) cinnamon chips

WHAT YOU'LL NEED

1-qt (1-L) jar

Strainer

Jar or bottle, for storage

Get outside and harvest your ingredients or purchase from a local organic farmer or herbalist.

Wash and dry the plants and roots to remove dirt. One by one, chop up all the herbs and roots and place them into a 1-quart (1-L) jar. Add any of the optional herbs that you'd like.

Once all the herbs have been added, if using honey, you can add it now. Fill the jar with apple cider vinegar and cover using either a BPA-free plastic lid or a layer of cheesecloth under a metal lid. Shake it well, then open the jar up and check to see if the vinegar level has dropped. If it has, add more vinegar to top it off and cover back up.

Label the jar and let sit for 4 to 6 weeks. Store in a place where you'll see it often. Shake it every week, taste a drop or two and keep it topped off with vinegar as needed. After 4 to 6 weeks, strain into a labeled jar or decorative bottle and enjoy.

TO USE
This blend tastes great added to a little bubbly water and sweetened with honey, enjoyed before or after a meal. It can be made into a salad dressing and essentially be used in any recipes calling for vinegar.

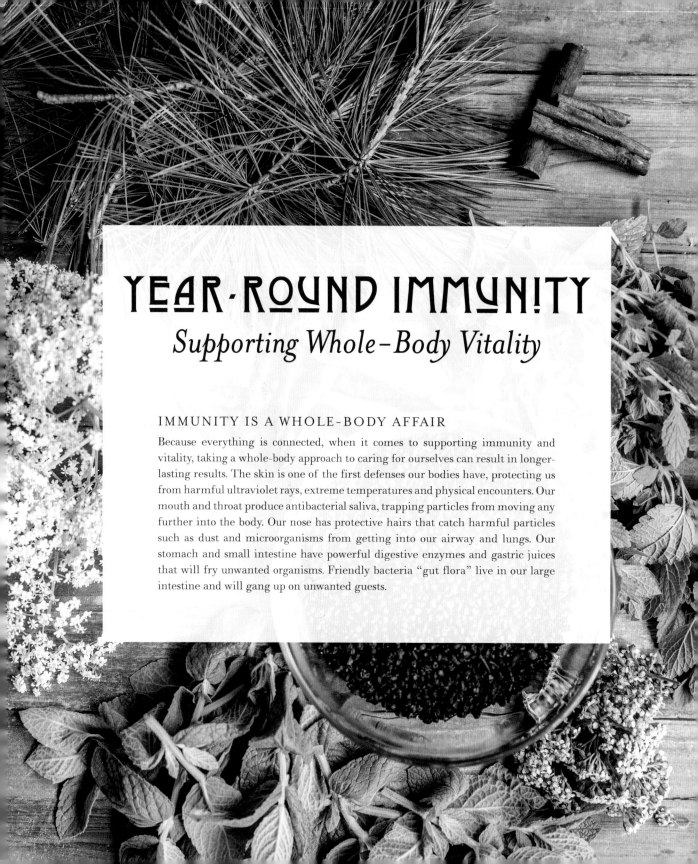

YEAR-ROUND IMMUNITY
Supporting Whole-Body Vitality

IMMUNITY IS A WHOLE-BODY AFFAIR

Because everything is connected, when it comes to supporting immunity and vitality, taking a whole-body approach to caring for ourselves can result in longer-lasting results. The skin is one of the first defenses our bodies have, protecting us from harmful ultraviolet rays, extreme temperatures and physical encounters. Our mouth and throat produce antibacterial saliva, trapping particles from moving any further into the body. Our nose has protective hairs that catch harmful particles such as dust and microorganisms from getting into our airway and lungs. Our stomach and small intestine have powerful digestive enzymes and gastric juices that will fry unwanted organisms. Friendly bacteria "gut flora" live in our large intestine and will gang up on unwanted guests.

Then there's the lymphatic system. Our lymph system is a major player in our immune health. It's where lymphocytes, also known as white blood cells, are produced; this is one of our body's top defense systems. Our lymphatic system runs throughout the entire body, working with the thymus, spleen, tonsils and lymphatic tissue. The lymphatic system moves lymph fluid passively throughout the body. The fluid collects between cells, drains into lymph vessels and then flows into our lymph nodes, which are little filtration and storage systems located throughout the body. When our bodies are fighting something, it's normal for these nodes to swell and be a little sore, which can be a warning sign that something is going on.

I want you to be able to visualize how the immune system runs throughout the entire body. If something is going on with our digestive system and there is an inflammatory response, then our immune system is involved. If we're stressed, we create a hormone called cortisol, which will suppress our immune system, making us more vulnerable to diseases and infections. I bet you've experienced this effect, like a time you were super stressed only to come out of it with a cold, flu or another illness or disease.

It's important to keep our body and immune system well supported year-round to enhance everyday vitality. Don't wait until you're sick. There are preventive things you can be doing. Start with the food you eat, by reducing sugar, dairy and processed foods, all of which can increase inflammation in the body. We want to eat a vitamin- and mineral-rich diet loaded with healthy and colorful vegetables and fruits—basically, we should be eating a rainbow. Stay hydrated with lots of water, limiting caffeine/coffee, soda and alcohol. Move your body. This is one of the best things for your immune and lymphatic system. This doesn't have to be marathon movement—a nice daily walk is great. Just get out and move every day. Other things that can be beneficial for our immune and lymph system are dry brushing, saunas and massage.

And of course, there are herbs. Many wonderful herbs help support our vitality and daily health. I would suggest adding adaptogens, such as mushrooms, to your daily routine. Mushrooms are a great way to support full-body vitality throughout the year. Here in Maine, we have a handful of amazing medicinal mushrooms that grow wild, such as belted polypore, maitake, reishi, lion's mane and chaga, and my favorite way to use these mushrooms is in foods and drinks. Of course, if these aren't available fresh where you are, you can buy them dried.

Elderberry is an amazing immune-supporting herb. Taking elderberries at the onset of cold or flu symptoms will help shorten the duration or ward it off. The constituents in elderberries encourage our body to create more fighter cells to go after invading viruses. They're also high in antioxidants, vitamin A, vitamin C and flavonoids, which can help prevent oxidative damage to cells. It's a lovely sour and tart little berry that I mostly make into an elixir, syrup or drinks and use throughout the cold and flu months.

Our respiratory system can get slammed when our immune system is working overtime, resulting in coughs, sneezing and excess mucus. So, it's always important to support the respiratory system with plenty of herbs that are expectorants, such as hyssop and mullein, which help break up and expel mucus. Marshmallow, another mucilaginous herb, is soothing and calming to inflamed tissue.

You also definitely want to have some antiviral and antimicrobial herbs in the mix, including thyme, rosemary and garlic. I would suggest incorporating garlic, onions, thyme and rosemary into your winter meals and enjoying some lemon balm ginger honey tea. It's a delicious way to enjoy food and drink while supporting your body with some fabulous antivirals.

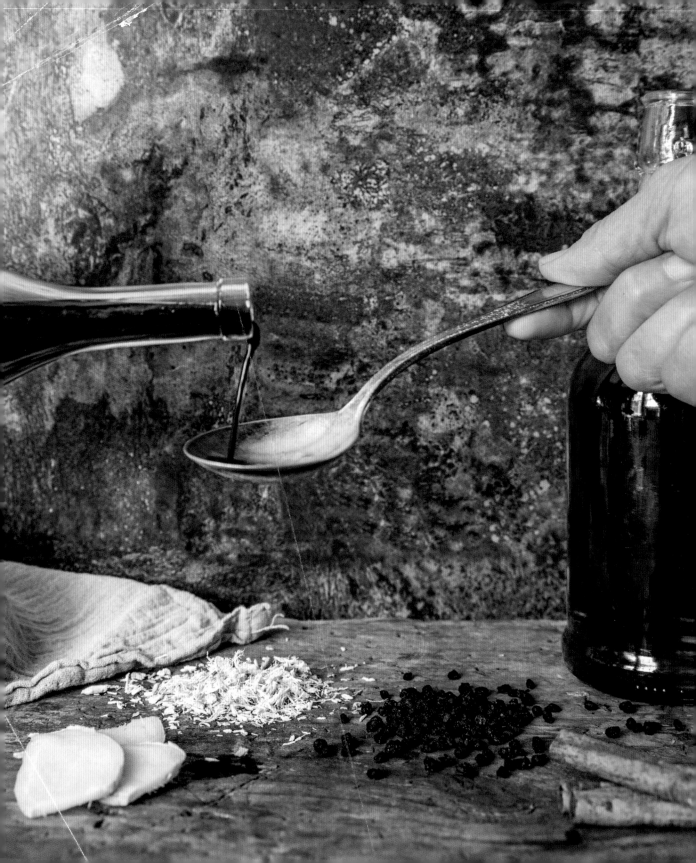

ELDERBERRY SYRUP WITH REISHI + ROOTS

Makes 2–3 cups (480–720 ml)

Elderberry is a must-have in the kitchen. These tart and sour berries pack a punch in helping our bodies stay vital and strong during the cold and flu season.

One winter, I was dealing with a weakened immune system due to Lyme disease. I decided I had had enough of getting sick every winter for weeks on end, so I formulated an elixir for myself. At the time I had not come across any formulas on the market blending medicinal mushrooms and immune-supporting roots with elderberry, and that's exactly what my body needed. Not only did that formula keep my immune system supported that winter, but it's also gone on to become our multi-award-winning Elderberry, Mushroom + Roots Elixir and one of our top-selling formulas.

I recommend you start using this blend daily September through May. Take a small spoonful or dropperful for preventive care. If you start to feel a cold, flu or illness come on, increase the dosage to a spoonful every couple of hours every day to help your body actively fight the illness.

INGREDIENTS

2 cups (236 g) dried elderberries

2–4 tsp (9–18 g) cinnamon chips

2–3 tsp (6–9 g) dried ginger pieces

2 tbsp (10 g) dried astragalus root

2 tbsp (5 g) dried sliced reishi pieces

4 cups (960 ml) cold water

1 tsp lemon juice

½–2 cups (160–640 g) honey
or maple syrup

1 cup (240 ml) vodka or brandy
(optional, to extend storage life)

WHAT YOU'LL NEED

3-qt (3-L) pot

Strainer

Sterilized bottles or jars,
for storage

Place the elderberries, cinnamon, ginger, astragalus, reishi and water in a pot and bring to a boil over high heat. When it reaches a boil, reduce the heat and simmer for about 40 minutes. You want to reduce the liquid by half (about 2 cups [480 ml]). Turn off the heat and let the mixture cool for about an hour, then strain.

Next add the lemon juice and sweetener. Using 2 cups (640 g) of sweetener will make the syrup more shelf-stable, but super sweet. So, if you're like me, use less sweetener (start with ½ cup [160 g], taste and adjust from there), then just store in the fridge. I go through it so fast it never lasts long enough to go bad. You could also add the optional alcohol and store in the fridge if you don't think you'll use it as often. When ready, bottle into labeled jars and store in the fridge.

TO USE

Take ½ to 1 teaspoon once per day as preventive care. Increase to taking ½ to 1 teaspoon multiple times a day if you feel something coming on.

GINGER + ELDERBERRY HOT TODDY WITH ELDERFLOWER BRANDY

Makes 2 cups (480 ml) Elderflower Brandy and 3 (¾-cup [180-ml]) servings Elderberry Hot Toddy

It's winter, there's snow on the ground and you just had a great time outside, but it's cold as hell out and you're ready to get cozy. A great way to warm up is with this tasty immune-supporting hot toddy that's made with elderberries, ginger and reishi mushroom—all herbs that support vitality and immune health. Ginger is warming and great for energizing circulation throughout the body. Reishi mushrooms are wonderful for restoring vital immune activity, especially in people who have been in a depleted state. This hot toddy is a delicious and fun way to add these immune-boosting herbs to your day.

First, you'll need to make some Elderflower Brandy. Elderflowers have a history of use as a remedy for colds and flu, and are especially used in fever tea blends. Elderflowers are antiviral, diaphoretic and anti-inflammatory. Best of all, they're delicious and make a super tasty brandy! I'd also suggest making the Elderberry Syrup with Reishi + Roots on page 61, which you can use in the toddy for sweetness and an extra boost.

ELDERFLOWER BRANDY
¼ cup (29 g) dried elderflowers

2 cups (480 ml) brandy

ELDERBERRY HOT TODDY
1–2 tbsp (8–16 g) grated fresh ginger

Zest from 1 lemon
(1–2 tbsp [6–12 g] zest)

2 tbsp (18 g) dried elderberries

1 tbsp (11 g) cinnamon chips or
1 cinnamon stick

2 tsp (8 g) dried reishi powder

4 cups (960 ml) water

1 tbsp (15 ml) lemon juice, divided

1½ tsp (7 ml) maple syrup or
Elderberry Syrup with Reishi +
Roots (page 61), divided

1½ tsp–3 tbsp (7–45 ml) Elderflower
Brandy (optional), divided

WHAT YOU'LL NEED
2 (16-oz [480-ml]) jars

Strainer

Microplane

3-qt (3-L) pot

TO MAKE THE ELDERFLOWER BRANDY
Place the dried elderflowers in a 16-ounce (480-ml) jar and pour in the brandy to the very top of the jar. Cover and let sit for 4 weeks. Strain into a second 16-ounce (480-ml) jar, label it and sip on its own or make into a hot toddy below.

TO MAKE THE ELDERBERRY HOT TODDY
Place the grated ginger and the lemon zest in a pot. Add the elderberries, cinnamon, reishi and water. Bring to a boil over high heat, then reduce the heat to low and simmer for 25 to 30 minutes. You're looking to reduce the mixture by about half. When reduced, remove from the heat and strain. You should have a little over 2 cups (480 ml) or so of liquid.

Divide the liquid among three serving cups, which should come out to just under ¾ cup (180 ml) of liquid in each cup. Add 1 teaspoon of the lemon juice and ½ teaspoon of the maple syrup to each cup and stir. If using, add ½ teaspoon to 1 tablespoon (15 ml) of the Elderflower Brandy. Cheers!

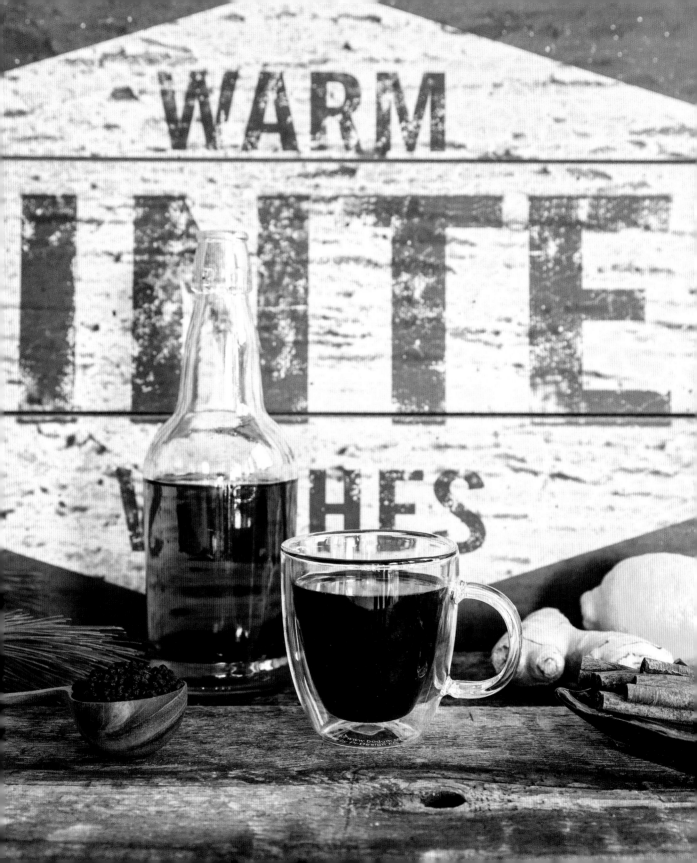

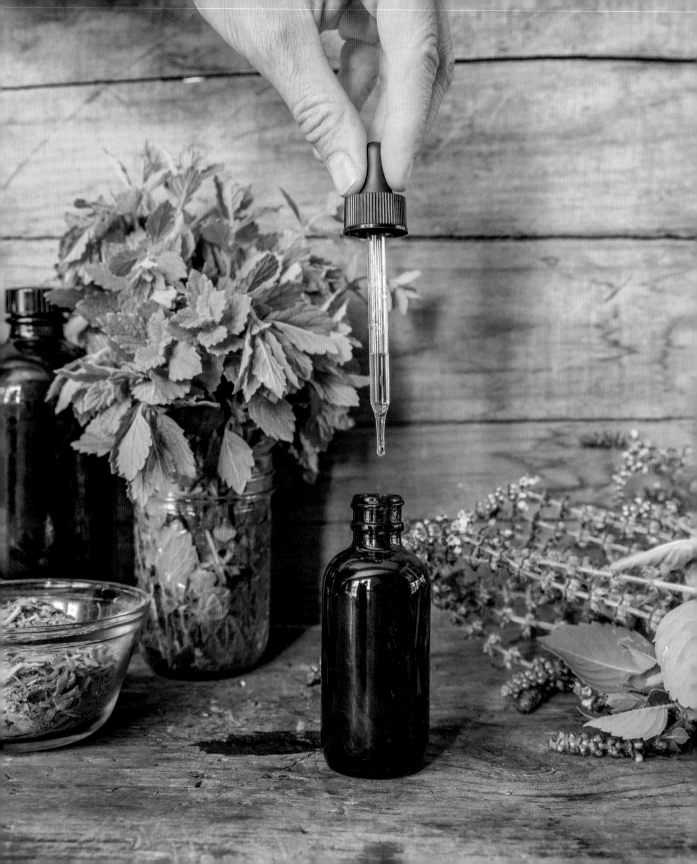

VITALITY TINCTURE

Makes 6–8 oz (180–240 ml)

When I think about vitality and immunity, I think about whole-body health. I carry this thought process into my formula blending. In this blend especially, you'll find a powerhouse combination of herbs to support immunity and vitality. Licorice root supports immune functions, soothes tissue in the upper respiratory tract and is a great anti-inflammatory and demulcent for the digestive tract. Lemon balm is a nervine and carminative and has antiviral activity, making it great for supporting the digestive, immune and nervous systems. Tulsi is a wonderful adaptogen and immune amphoteric that can help support and restore immune vitality. A good time to start making this blend is in late summer so it's ready by fall for the cold and flu season.

INGREDIENTS
2 tbsp (3 g) dried lemon balm

1 tbsp (3 g) dried tulsi

1 tbsp (9 g) dried ashwagandha

2 tsp (9 g) dried cinnamon chips

1 tsp dried licorice root (see Note)

2 tsp (13 g) honey (optional)

About 1 cup (240 ml) vodka

WHAT YOU'LL NEED
Spice grinder

8-oz (240-ml) jar

Strainer

4 (2-oz [60-ml]) dropper bottles or a jar, for storage

When making medicine, holding intent and vision is an important part of the process. As you're gathering your herbs, meditate on why you're making this tincture, whether it's for yourself, a family member or a friend in need. Hold your reasons for making this medicine close to you while going through the following steps.

Gather your herbs and one by one, measure them out and run them through a spice grinder, then place into an 8-ounce (240-ml) jar. If you don't have a grinder you can just measure out the herbs and place directly into the jar.

Once all the herbs are in the jar, if using honey, you can add it now. Next, pour in the vodka until the jar is filled. Mix it all together and add more alcohol if needed, then place the cap on and shake. Open the jar back up and check to see if the alcohol level has dropped. If it has, add more to the jar and cover back up.

Label your jar and let sit for 4 weeks. Store in a place where you'll see it often. Shake it every week and taste a drop or two. After 4 weeks, strain and bottle in labeled 2-ounce (60-ml) dropper bottles or a jar.

TO USE
Take 1 to 2 full droppers (¼ to ½ teaspoon), in water or tea, one to three times a day. I recommend taking daily during the fall, winter and early spring.

Note: Omit licorice root from the formula if you have hypertension, congestive heart failure, edema, hyperkalemia or kidney disease. Omit it if you are taking digoxin, MAOIs, SSRIs, diuretics, antihypertensives or anticoagulants.

FEVER BREAK TEA + BATH

Makes 2⅛ cups (105 g) herb blend

Fevers are a quick indicator that our bodies are actively fighting something off. Although it's an important process, it can be an uncomfortable one, especially if the body is struggling to sweat it out. The base of this tea blend is a true classic, and for good reason. It comes through time and time again. Many of the herbs in this blend are diuretics, such as yarrow, mint and elderflower, which help us sweat the fever out. I also like to add white pine needles to support the lungs and add some vitamin C, as well as boneset for aches and pain. Hopefully you, your family and friends won't need this one often, but if you do, I hope it helps you feel better soon! Also, this blend can be used in the bath, and I've given instructions for using it that way below.

TEA + BATH

½ cup (60 g) dried elderflower

½ cup (10 g) dried yarrow

½ cup (23 g) dried mint

¼ cup (27 g) dried rose hips

¼ cup (12 g) fresh or dried
white pine needles

2 tbsp (4 g) dried boneset

OPTIONAL ADDITIONS (FOR TEA)

2 tbsp (18 g) grated fresh ginger

Lemon wedge

Honey, to taste

WHAT YOU'LL NEED

16-oz (480-ml) jar

Kettle

Strainer

5" x 7" (13 x 18–cm) muslin bag
(for bath)

TO MAKE THE HERB BLEND

Gather your herbs in a mixing bowl. Blend with your hands until it all comes together. Store in a jar to use as needed.

TO MAKE THE TEA

To make a cup of tea, use 1½ teaspoons (1.5 g) of the herb blend to 1 cup (240 ml) of boiling water. Add the ginger, a squeeze from the lemon wedge and honey, if desired. Let sit for 5 to 10 minutes. Strain the herbs and enjoy. Drink 1 to 3 cups (240 to 720 ml) a day at the onset of a fever, until the fever has gone down.

TO MAKE THE BATH

Fill the muslin bag with 2 to 4 tablespoons (6 to 12 g) of the blend, close the bag and add it to your bath. Or you could also make a pot of tea using all of the herb blend, then strain and add to the bathwater. This is often how I do it when I want it to be a stronger bath.

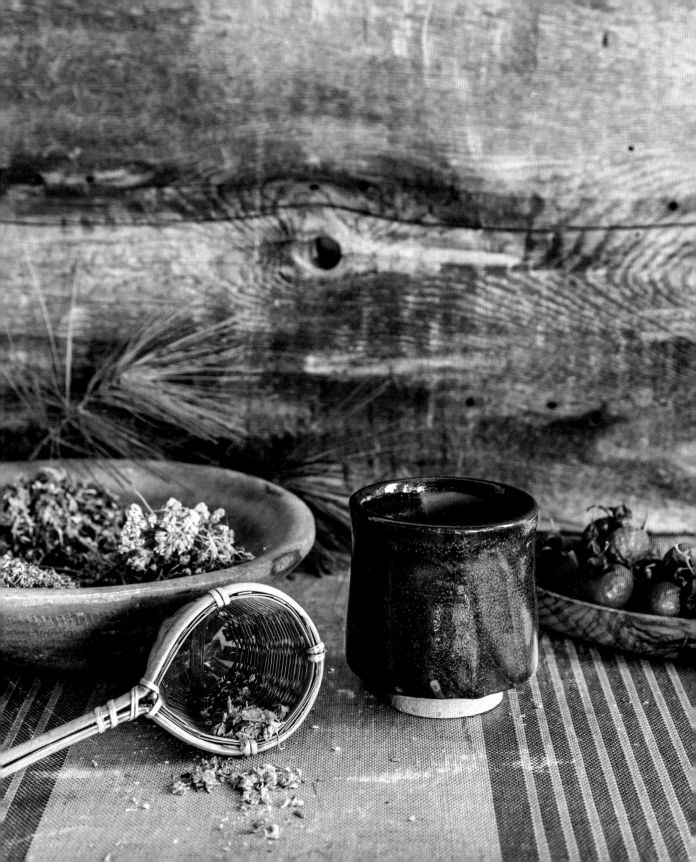

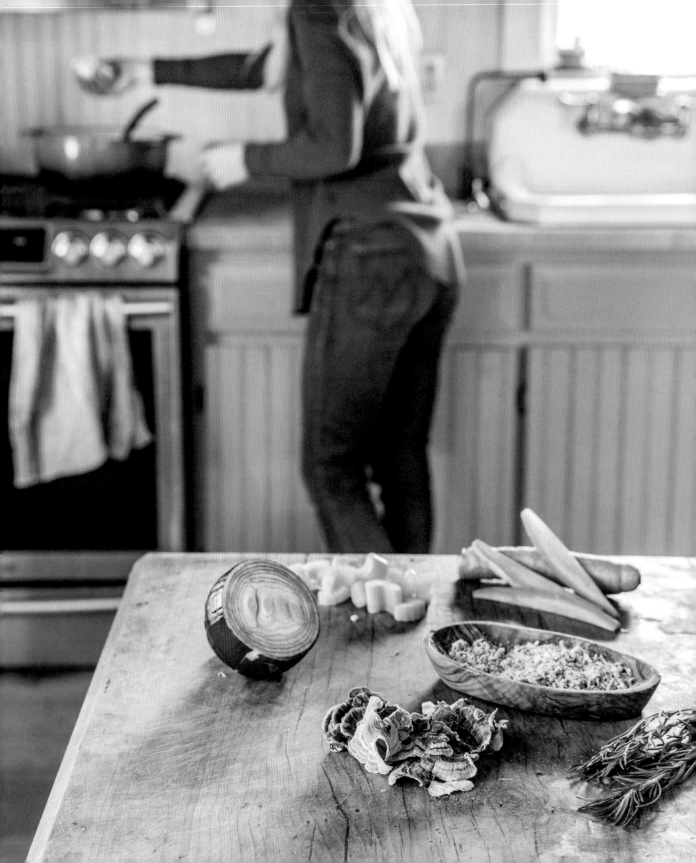

MEDICINAL MUSHROOM SOUP STOCK

Makes 4–6 cups (960 ml–1.4 L)

Mushrooms are a fabulous way to support our immune, upper respiratory and cardiovascular systems. They are anti-inflammatory, antiviral, high in antioxidants and so much more. One of my favorite ways to work with mushrooms is through food. Some delicious edible medicinal mushrooms include—but are certainly not limited to— lion's mane, maitake and shiitake. There are a number of other medicinal mushrooms that are hard and woody, such as reishi, turkey tail and chaga. The best way to add these mushrooms to your diet is in a decoction, reduction sauce or, one of my favorites, soup stock such as this one. It's important to cook mushrooms to help break down their cell walls to access the medicinal polysaccharides, making soup stocks a great way to utilize the benefits of the herbs and mushroom while knowing you're offering your body incredible nourishment.

When making soup stock, I add lots of other immune-supporting herbs such as astragalus, codonopsis, burdock root, rosemary, thyme and garlic. I also like to add whatever veggies I have in the house that day. If you're not a vegetarian, you can also throw in some bones. You can truly tailor this however you like.

STOCK

⅓–½ cup (12–18 g) dried reishi (pieces or slices)

⅓–½ cup (12–18 g) dried maitake

2 tbsp (9 g) dried astragalus root

2 tbsp (22 g) dried burdock root

1 whole garlic bulb, cloves peeled and smashed

1 medium onion, roughly chopped

2 celery ribs with leaves, roughly chopped

1 cup (66 g) kale or kale ribs, roughly chopped

3 qt (3 L) water

OPTIONAL ADDITIONS

2 tbsp (15 g) codonopsis root

2–4 tbsp (5–10 g) dried nettle

¼ cup (6 g) dried milky oat tops

2 tbsp (7 g) dried rosemary

2 tbsp (7 g) dried thyme

2 tbsp (5 g) dried oregano

1–2 tbsp (9–18 g) grated fresh ginger

2 tsp (6 g) dried turmeric

2 carrots

WHAT YOU'LL NEED

Large pot

Strainer

3 (1-pint [480-ml]) or 2 (1-qt [1-L]) sterile jars, for storage

Ice cube trays

Place everything in the pot and bring to a boil over high heat, then reduce the heat and cook at a nice steady simmer for at least 4 hours and up to 6 hours. You will most likely need to add more water to the pot as the water reduces, but ultimately you are looking to yield about 6 cups (1.4 L) of stock after 4 hours of simmering.

When the stock is done cooking, strain well and store in labeled jars. You can then use the stock as a base for any recipe calling for broth or stock. The fresh stock will keep for 5 days in the fridge, and up to 12 months in the freezer.

I like to freeze my stock in 1-pint (480-ml) and 1-quart (1-L) jars. I fill hot sterile jars about three-fourths of the way with the stock and then let them cool on the counter. Once cool, I place them in the freezer without a top. Once they're frozen, I place a cover on the jars and label the lid.

You can also freeze some of the stock in ice cube trays. When frozen, remove from the tray and store in a freezer bag in the freezer. The ice cubes are great to add to tea, make into miso soup, deglaze pans and so on. Another great option is to use the stock to cook grains.

Note: For more mycological inspiration, check out Paul Stamets at Fungi.com and books by Christopher Hobbs.

FIRE CIDER

Makes 4 cups (960 ml)

Fire cider is a wonderful kitchen remedy created by Rosemary Gladstar back in the late 1970s. It's incredibly versatile and can be used to improve energy and boost the immune system, especially when you feel something coming on. It also supports the upper respiratory and circulatory systems, and helps with allergies, heartburn/ acid reflux and aching joints. To this day fire cider remains a beloved traditional herbal product.

In recent years, the herbal community was rocked by a controversy around fire cider. In 2012, a company called Shire City Herbals trademarked the name fire cider. The herbal community was outraged and responded with boycotts and petitions to cancel the trademark with the U.S. Patent and Trademark office. Subsequently, Shire City sued me and two other herbalists, Nicole Telkes and Mary Blue, for trademark infringement. In the spring of 2019, the case went to trial in federal court. The incredible support of Rosemary, our lawyers, family and the herbal community helped us stand strong, and in October of 2019, we received the much anticipated verdict . . . WE WON! This verdict was an incredible accomplishment for the herbal community, and today I'm honored to share my interpretation of Rosemary's classic method with you in this book.

CIDER

½ cup (72 g) grated fresh horseradish

⅓ cup (36 g) grated fresh ginger

1 large red or yellow onion

5–10 cloves garlic, smashed

1–3 fresh hot peppers, such as jalapeños, cayenne or habanero

2–4 tbsp (40–80 g) honey, or more to taste

4 cups (960 ml) raw apple cider vinegar

OPTIONAL ADDITIONS

Oranges and/or lemons

Turmeric

Elderberries

Hyssop

Bee Balm

Rosemary and/or thyme

WHAT YOU'LL NEED

Grater or food processor

1-qt (1-L) jar

Strainer

Bottles or jar, for storage

When grating the horseradish and ginger, you can use a traditional box grater or run them through the grater on a food processor. Be aware, the fumes from grating horseradish can be intense and can burn—think wasabi.

Place the horseradish and ginger in the jar. Chop the onion, garlic and hot peppers or run through the food processor with the shredding attachment, then place in the jar.

At this point, you can add whatever extra ingredients you would like and the honey. Fill the jar completely with the raw apple cider vinegar, label the jar, then cover and allow it to infuse. For best results, you'll want to let this sit for at least 4 to 6 weeks. Store it in a place where you'll see it and shake it every week. After 4 to 6 weeks, strain the liquid into a clean labeled quart jar or bottles and enjoy!

I love using fire cider all on its own, but I also love making things with it. I make all my own salad dressings, so I use this for the vinegar. I love adding it to soups or roasted veggies, or making it into a drink (such as the Rise + Shine Tonic on page 72).

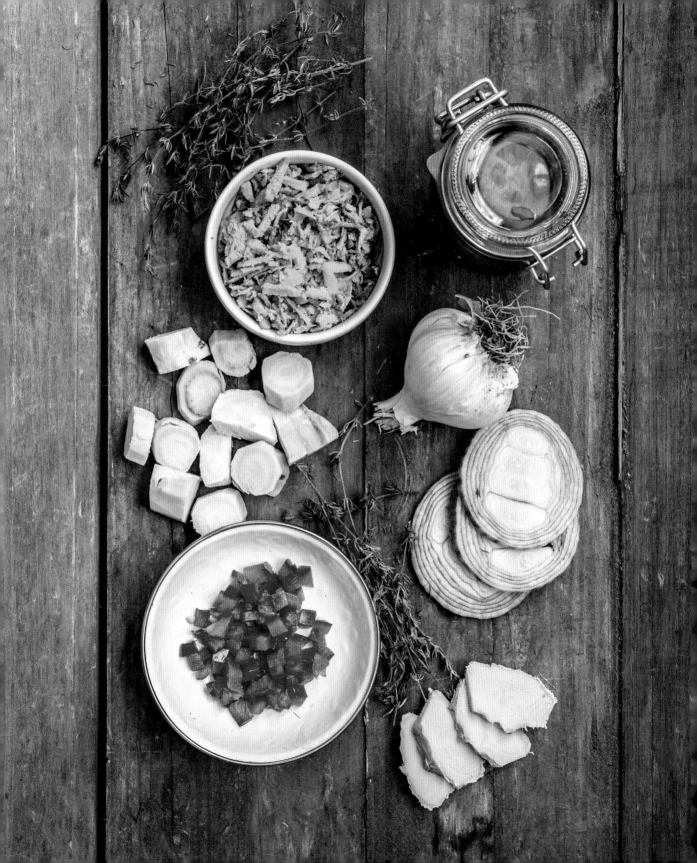

RISE + SHINE TONIC

Makes 1 serving

This is a great use for Fire Cider (page 70) that we like to take in the morning to get our day shaking!

INGREDIENTS

1 tbsp (15 ml) Fire Cider (page 70)

1 tbsp (15 ml) fresh squeezed orange juice

¼ cup (60 ml) sparkling or still water

¼ tsp honey, or to taste

Combine the cider, orange juice, water and honey in a jar or glass. Shake or stir well to mix up, and enjoy!

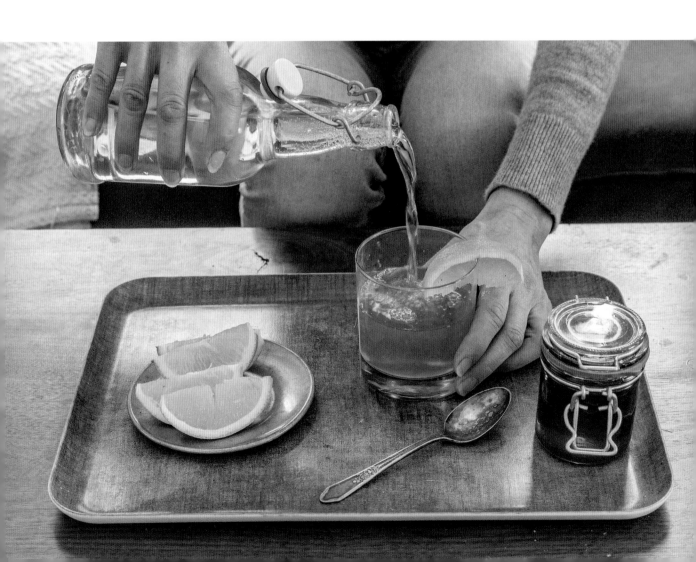

BREATHE DEEP RESPIRATORY TEA

Yield varies

Our respiratory system can take a beating in the wintertime with all the viruses floating around and the drying, cold air. This tea is a great one to have on hand in case you start to get that tickle in the back of your throat or are already in the midst of congestion. Marshmallow, plantain and lemon balm are relaxing to the upper respiratory tract. They are expectorants and soothing demulcents. Marshmallow is wonderfully cooling for hot and inflamed tissue in the respiratory system, and plantain leaf can be soothing for a dry and irritated throat. Lemon balm is antiviral, antimicrobial and a mild antispasmodic. This is just the thing to have in the pantry ready to go for when your upper respiratory tract is in despair.

INGREDIENTS

3 parts dried lemon balm

2 parts dried plantain leaf

2 parts dried marshmallow root

2 parts dried hyssop

1 part dried licorice root

WHAT YOU'LL NEED

Jar, for storage

Kettle

Strainer

First decide how much of the tea blend you'd like to make. I typically use cups for the parts so I have a large batch that will last me a few weeks or longer. If you'd like a smaller amount, use tablespoons, or use teaspoons for a single cup. Tablespoon measurements will give you a little over ½ cup (33 g) of tea blend. If using cups, you'll get about 10 cups (665 g) tea blend.

Once you've chosen your measurements, gather the herbs and measure them layer by layer into a mixing bowl. Blend together and store in a jar.

To make a cup of tea, use 1½ to 2 teaspoons (2 to 3 g) of tea blend to 1 cup (240 ml) of boiling water. Steep for 10 to 30 minutes, then strain into a cup and enjoy.

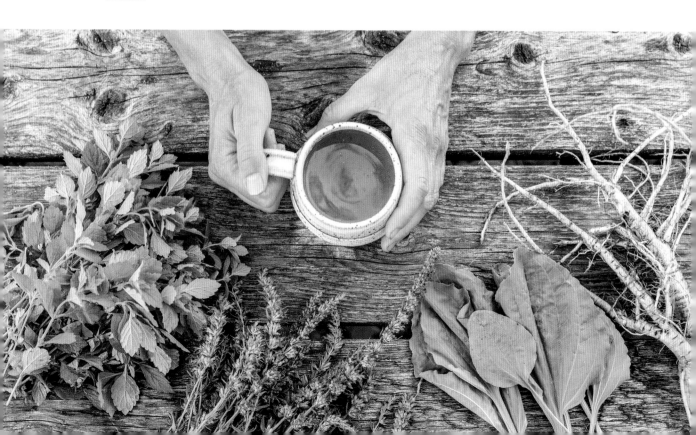

HEY HONEY

Makes 8 oz (225 g)

Honey is a fun and delicious way to work with herbs. Raw honey on its own is antibacterial, antifungal, high in antioxidants, prebiotic and packed with phyto-nutrients, and there is research to suggest that 2 teaspoons (14 g) of honey is better than over-the-counter medications for sore throats and coughs. All great reasons to combine it with herbs to make medicinal honeys.

When making herbal honey, I tend to use a lot of antiviral, antimicrobial and immune-supporting herbs such as hyssop, rosemary, lemon and garlic. This recipe and Keep Talking Honey on page 77 can both be used to soothe sore throats, coughs and the upper respiratory tract. Medicinal honeys are also a great way to introduce kids to using herbs, and they're fun and easy to make with them.

INGREDIENTS

1 cup (320 g) raw honey, divided

2 (¼" [6-mm]-thick) slices fresh red onion

1 clove garlic, smashed

2–4 thin slices fresh ginger

1 tsp dried hyssop

2 slices fresh lemon

WHAT YOU'LL NEED

8-oz (240-ml) jar

Strainer

Bottle, for storage

Pour a small layer of honey into the bottom of an 8-ounce (240-ml) jar. Add the red onion, then pour another thin layer of honey on top of the red onion slices. Next, cover the honey layer with a smashed clove of garlic, then another layer of honey. Repeat the layering process with the thinly sliced ginger, the dried hyssop and lastly the lemon slices, making sure to add a layer of honey between each addition.

Place the jar on the counter in a warm or sunny spot and let it infuse for 5 to 12 days, then strain the honey and store in a labeled bottle in the fridge. I like to eat the strained garlic, ginger and onions. You also don't need to strain.

TO USE

Take the medicinal honey straight by the spoonful to help ward off colds and flu. It's also great added to warm water, tea, salad dressings and sauces.

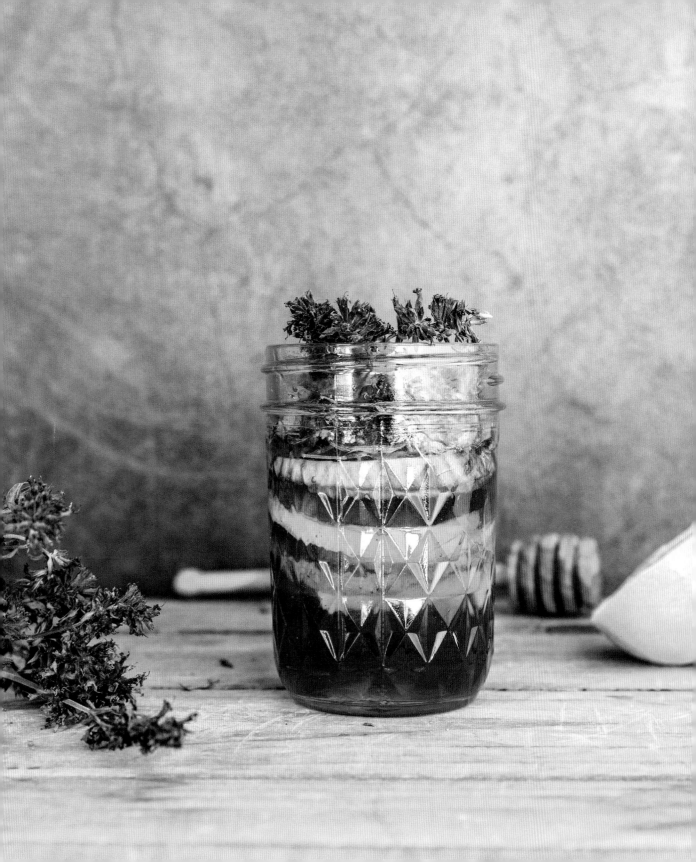

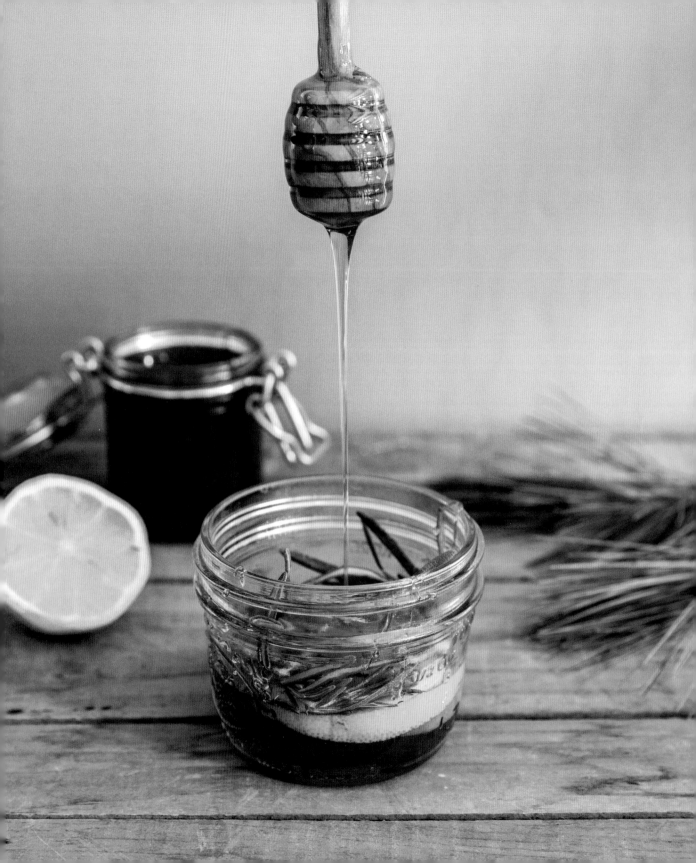

KEEP TALKING HONEY

Makes 6–8 oz (170–225 g)

I love having this on hand for sore throats and coughs, but I especially enjoy it when I'm working events and talking to thousands of people. My throat gets hoarse and sore, and I've even lost my voice for a short period! So, it's important for me to have this honey to help soothe my throat. If you find yourself with a hoarse and sore throat, this is definitely an herbal medicine you will want to have on hand. Even better, the flavors are absolutely delicious together.

INGREDIENTS

Raw honey as needed to fill the jar

4 (¼" [6-mm]) slices fresh lemon, divided

2 tsp (2 g) dried rosemary

2 (¼" [6-mm]) slices fresh ginger

2 tbsp (6 g) fresh or dried white pine needles

WHAT YOU'LL NEED

8-oz (240-ml) jar

Strainer

Bottle, for storage

Pour a small layer of honey in the bottom of the jar. Then add 2 slices of the lemon over the honey and pour another thin layer of honey on top of the lemon. Next, add a layer of rosemary and another thin layer of honey over that. Then add a layer of ginger slices and cover with a layer of honey. Now add the white pine layer and cover that with honey. Finally, add the remaining 2 lemon slices and cover that with honey.

Place the jar on the counter in a warm or sunny spot and let it infuse for 5 to 12 days. Strain the honey into a labeled bottle and store in the fridge.

TO USE

Take the medicinal honey straight by the spoonful to soothe the throat, or add to warm water, tea or syrups.

LOVE YOUR LYMPH TINCTURE + TEA

Makes 6–8 oz (180–240 ml) tincture,
½ cup (28 g) loose-leaf tea

There are a handful of things that we can do to support our lymphatic system. Moving our bodies is a great way to stimulate the lymphatic system. Self-care practices such as massage, dry brushing, taking a bath, using a sauna and using herbs are also beneficial. The formula below has some of my favorite lymph-loving herbs, such as calendula, cleaver and echinacea. This is a great blend to take if you're feeling lymph stagnation or swollen lymph glands. The herbs in this blend are anti-inflammatory, cleansing, detoxing, immune enhancing and lymph stimulating. You can make this into a tea or a tincture. Your choice.

INGREDIENTS

3 tbsp (3 g) dried calendula

2 tbsp (6 g) dried cleavers

2 tbsp (3 g) dried red clover blossoms

1 tbsp (11 g) dried burdock root
or dandelion root

1 tbsp (5 g) dried echinacea

1 cup (240 ml) vodka (for tincture)

WHAT YOU'LL NEED

Spice grinder (for tincture)

8-oz (240-ml) jar

Strainer

4 (2-oz [60-ml]) dropper bottles or
a jar (for tincture)

Kettle

TO MAKE THE TINCTURE

Gather your herbs and one by one, measure them out and run them through a spice grinder, then place into an 8-ounce (240-ml) jar. If you don't have a grinder, you can just measure out the herbs and place directly into the jar.

Stir the herbs around in the jar and add vodka to top off the jar. Then place the cap on and shake. Open the jar back up and check to see if the alcohol level has dropped. If it has, add more to the jar and cover back up.

Label the jar and let sit for 4 weeks. Store in a place where you'll see it often. Shake it every week and taste a drop or two. After 4 weeks, you can strain and bottle into labeled 2-ounce (60-ml) dropper bottles or a jar.

TO USE

Take 1 to 2 full droppers (¼ to ½ teaspoon) one to three times a day.

TO MAKE THE TEA

Gather the herbs and blend them together in a bowl. Store them in an 8-ounce (240-ml) jar and use as needed.

Use 1½ teaspoons (2 g) per 1 cup (240 ml) of boiling water. Steep for 10 to 20 minutes, then strain into a cup and enjoy. Drink 1 to 2 cups (240 to 480 ml) a day as needed.

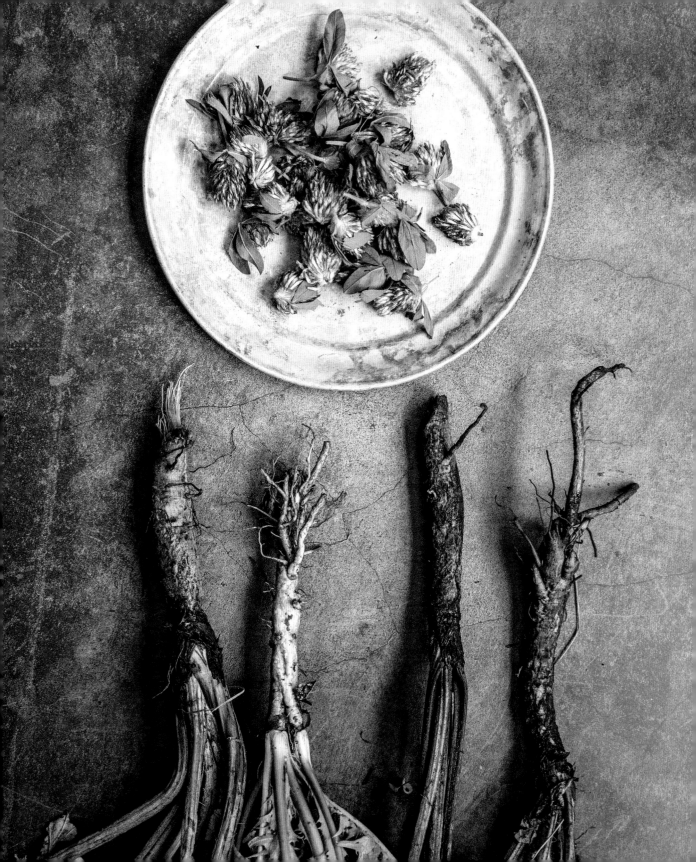

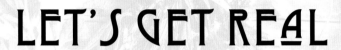

LET'S GET REAL
Women's Health + Sexuality

THE LEGACY OF WOMEN HERBALISTS

Women throughout the centuries have played their roles both at the front of the line and behind it. History is rich with women being persecuted to death for their knowledge of plants, herbal medicine and women's health and midwifery. This did not stop them. These women continued to learn the language of the plants, passing it on to the next generation. This knowledge is just as important and relevant today, where women are still fighting for their rights and access to proper health and birth care. As a woman, I'm thankful on a daily basis for all the women in the past who came before me fighting for women's rights and the women of today who stand strong, demanding the injustices be heard and who continue the radical act of learning and teaching the tradition of herbal knowledge.

Women throughout history and up to the present have dealt with sexual objectification, sexual persecution, sexual violence and shame. Around the globe women carry deep wounds caused by sexual trauma. Until now, most of these things weren't openly spoken about, and even today it's a challenge. Yet, more and more people are starting to recognize how many women are out there who have experienced sexual abuse and trauma. How many women have pushed down these traumas? As women, we have always turned to each other and to plants. As herbalists, it's important for us to recognize and hold the space that's required for this work. Working with herbs that support the nervous system is key here: herbs that bring a sense of comfort, peace and safety, such as rose, milky oat tops and lemon balm; herbs that can help ease panic and anxiety, such as blue vervain, motherwort and skullcap; and herbs that can help induce sleep, such as hops, passionflower and lavender.

HARNESSING THE POWER

Like the ocean's tide, our bodies, our cycles and our moods wax and wane with the moon. As we swell, our connection with water and moon energies strengthens as our intuition becomes more enhanced. Our senses heighten and we speak what we see and feel without our filters on. Our cycles can be a powerful time of the month for us, as we tap into a higher power of wisdom and knowledge. Our bodies are going through the same process they have since the beginning of time. We carry the layers and weight of history from the centuries of shame and persecution for this power, but we're in a time where women are reclaiming their bodies and sexuality and harnessing the mystical powers of our cycles.

Unfortunately, our cycles aren't usually about having sudden powers. They can mean extreme fatigue, dread, depression, fear, anxiety, self-doubt, major mood swings, bloating, weight gain, back pain, headaches, insomnia, painful cramps, excessive blood loss . . . should I go on? No doubt you are familiar with many of these symptoms, which can leave us feeling frustrated, annoyed and far from mystical.

There are a lot of amazing herbs that can help support us during these times—especially vitex berry, cramp bark, burdock and motherwort. Watching the foods we eat is always helpful as well. This can be challenging because we tend to crave everything under the sun, but if possible, try to cut back on refined, processed foods, especially white sugar and dairy products.

A lot of the hormones need to be processed through our liver, so to help ease some symptoms it can be beneficial to drink teas and take tinctures that are supportive to the liver and endocrine system—herbs such as dandelion root, burdock root and astragalus root.

MISCARRIAGES AND ABORTIONS

A miscarriage is something many women will experience and endure at least once in their lifetime, yet most friends and family will never know. The Mayo Clinic reports that 10 to 20 percent of known pregnancies end in miscarriage, yet this information is rarely discussed. As for abortions, women for the most part stay silent. There is great judgment and shame placed on women who make this decision. Women need support and understanding. There are many reasons women have abortions, and for many this can be a heart-wrenching decision. As someone that has experienced an abortion and numerous miscarriages, one almost resulting in my death, I feel compelled to speak out against the silence and shame. I encourage women to share with one another if they feel moved to and to encourage others to stop and listen from the heart, instead of placing shame and judgment.

It can be hard to see through the deep heartbreak, pain and shame of these experiences. Listening and talking to other women who have experienced miscarriages and abortions can help us build back strength in our hearts, bodies and minds and be there for others as they navigate their personal experience with their loss. It's important to allow ourselves time to process. If you can, I suggest reaching out to a support system of friends and family. If this is not an option, then consider reaching out to local midwives, Planned Parenthood, doula groups, clinical herbalists or NDs focused on women's health.

During this time, it's important to support the body with nourishing and nutritive herbs and to use flower essences to support the emotions. Rest as much as you can and eat warming, nourishing foods, such as soups and soup stocks with nettles, astragalus and mushrooms; dark leafy greens; and other easily digestible foods. Stay well hydrated and drink lots of warming nutritive infusions with herbs such as nettles, raspberry leaf, lemon balm, alfalfa, rose, tulsi and mint.

MENOPAUSE

As if the changes we experienced with puberty weren't enough, now we have to experience major hormonal changes again when our bodies start to go through perimenopause and menopause. We know we've reached menopause when we go twelve or more months without a menstrual cycle. Premenopause or perimenopause can start to happen in our late thirties and for some even twenties, but it's most typical for it to begin in our forties.

Perimenopause is the decline in ovarian production and can last for ten years as our bodies slowly stop producing sex hormones. Slowly, over time, our levels of estrogen and progesterone, both of which are produced by our ovaries, decrease. This change in our hormones, especially estrogen, can be troublesome and cause unpleasant symptoms, such as depression, hot flashes, low sex drive, vaginal dryness, insomnia, weight gain, mood swings, tender breasts, headaches and more.

Of course—always think about the foods you're consuming, where they come from and how they were raised. Get plenty of fruits, veggies and foods high in calcium, iron, protein and vitamin E and keep all processed food and junk food to a minimum. Drink a lot of water and tea, always, and make sure to get a little exercise in daily.

And, of course there are some herbs that can help support us as well, such as vitex berry, milky oat tops, blue vervain and motherwort. Also, there are herb books dedicated to perimenopause and menopause. Refer to the book list in the back for suggested reads.

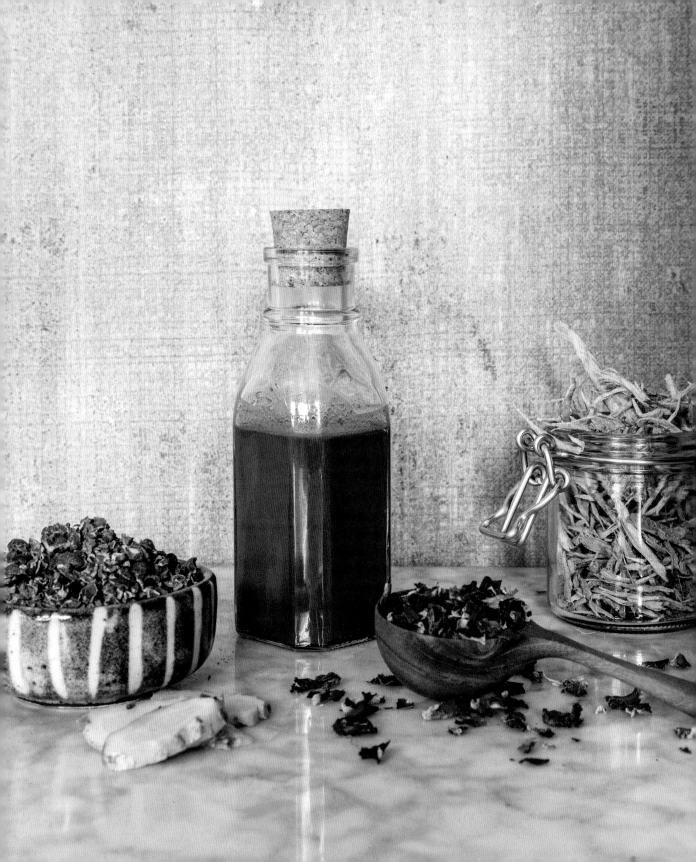

TRIPLE X CHOCOLATE LOVE CORDIAL

Makes 6–8 oz (180–240 ml)

Sensuality looks different for us all and may be harder to explore based on our life experiences. Sensuality is about exploring ourselves, learning what our desires are on a physical, emotional and even spiritual level. It's about understanding OUR desires, not the desires that someone else or society places upon us. This delicious blend made with chocolate, rose and ashwagandha can bring us inward, nourishing us and helping us heal and explore our sensual selves.

Rose has a long history of being connected with the heart, love and sensuality. Visually, it's beautiful and the smell is deeply sensual and intoxicating. Rose energetically offers love, support and guidance to help us explore deeper within ourselves, awakening our desires. Ashwagandha is a nourishing herb and adaptogen. I love using ashwagandha for nourishing the heart and reproductive system and for its history as an aphrodisiac. A high-quality bar of dark chocolate can change our mood, uplift our spirits, bring a sense of joy and make us feel like a high priestess or queen. Cacao has a high concentration of a chemical constituent called phenylethylamine, which is the same chemical produced in our brain when we feel love. This is why we get a lovely blissed-out feeling from eating chocolate.

INGREDIENTS

2 tbsp (17 g) raw cacao powder

2 tbsp (2 g) dried rose petals

2 tsp (6 g) dried ginger pieces

2 tsp (6 g) dried shatavari powder

1 tsp dried cinnamon powder

1 tsp dried ashwagandha powder

2 heaping tbsp (40 g) honey

Dash of vanilla extract (optional)

About 1 cup (240 ml) brandy

WHAT YOU'LL NEED

Spice grinder

8-oz (240-ml) jar

Strainer

4 (2-oz [60-ml]) dropper bottles or a jar, for storage

Gather your herbs and one by one, measure them out and run them through a spice grinder, then place into an 8-ounce (240-ml) jar. If you don't have a grinder, you can just measure out the herbs and place directly into the jar.

Next, add the honey and vanilla (if using). Then, fill the jar with brandy. Mix it all together and add more alcohol if needed to top off the jar. Then place the cap on and shake. Open the jar back up and check to see if the alcohol level has dropped. If it has, add more to the jar and cover back up.

Label your jar and let sit for 4 weeks. Store in a place where you'll see it often. Shake it every week and taste a drop or two. After 4 weeks, you can strain and bottle into labeled 2-ounce (60-ml) dropper bottles or a jar.

TO USE

Take 2 full droppers (½ teaspoon) one to three times a day. You can take it straight or add it to coffee, hot cacao or the Roasted Roots Herbal Coffee on page 24. You could also use it to make cocktails or mocktails. Have fun with it!

SENSUAL SIPPING CHOCOLATE WITH ROSE

Makes 4–6 servings

Throughout history, rose and chocolate have been renowned for their allure and sensuality. Stimulating our senses through beauty, taste and smell, roses and chocolate have a way of uplifting and setting the mood. This blend is more than just chocolate and roses, though; herbs such as ashwagandha, maca and shatavari have a history of use for enhancing female and male sexuality. Meeeow. Also, this blend is seriously delicious and can be enjoyed alone, with a partner or with a group of partners.

INGREDIENTS
2 tbsp (17 g) raw cacao powder

1 tsp maca powder

1 tsp dried rose petals

¾ tsp cinnamon powder

½ tsp shatavari powder

¼ tsp ashwagandha powder

Pinch of salt

Coconut milk or liquid of choice (see Notes)

Vanilla extract, to taste

Maple syrup, to taste

WHAT YOU'LL NEED
Spice grinder

8-oz (240-ml) storage jar

Pot

Strainer

Gather your herbs. If some of the herbs you can't find already powdered, you can purchase pieces and use the grinder to powder them yourself; just be sure to measure after grinding to get the right amount.

Place all of the powdered herbs and a pinch of salt into a bowl and blend well. Store the blend in a jar for later use or use right away.

TO USE
Use 1½ to 2 teaspoons (4 to 6 g) of the chocolate herb blend per 1 cup (240 ml) of coconut milk. Heat the milk with the chocolate herb blend in a pot on the stove over low heat for about 5 minutes, until warm.

To serve, add a drop of vanilla extract and a little maple syrup. You can strain if you like, but I usually don't. Enjoy!

Notes: If you don't like coconut milk, you can substitute with regular milk or any milk alternative. You could use any ratio of water to milk, cream or milk alternative. Maybe you want no water and all milk or cream.

A little nip of brandy tastes really good with this blend, or better yet, a rose vanilla brandy. Oh yeah.

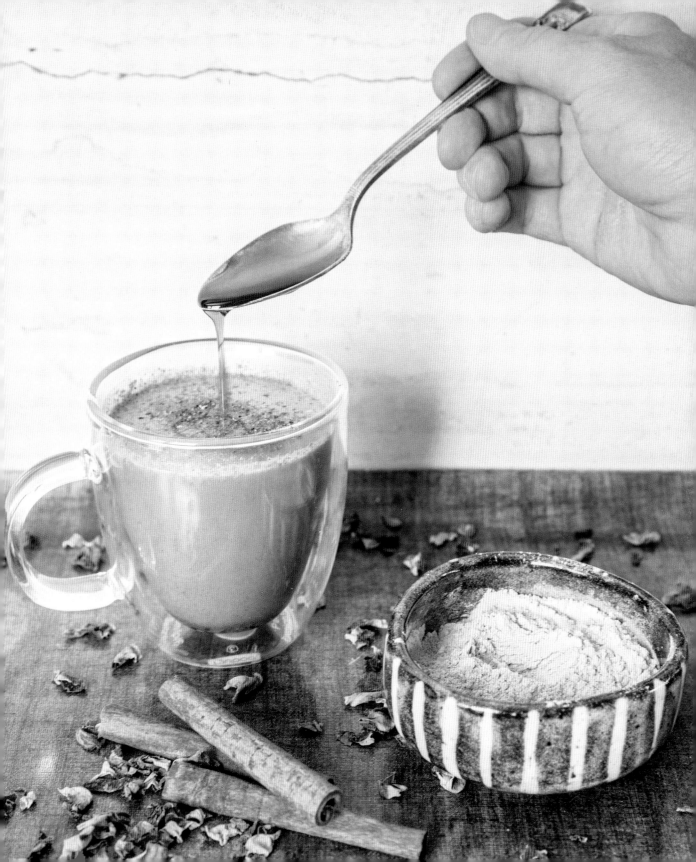

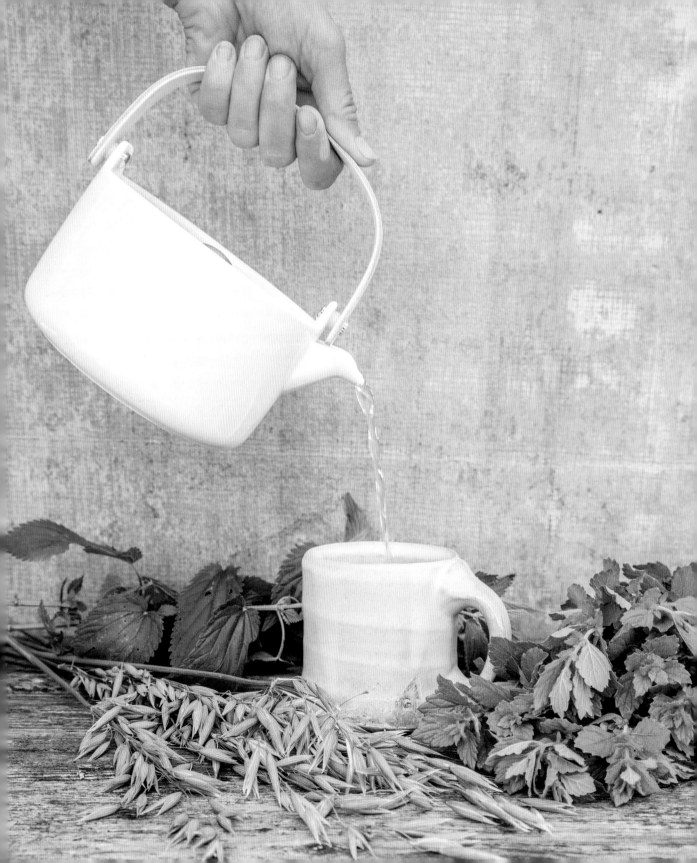

KEEP YOUR COOL INFUSION + TEA

Yield varies

Making tea can be a wonderful way to help calm your nerves, whether you're feeling anxious or irritable. The process of making tea takes time and patience. During the course of making the tea I often find that I've processed whatever was bothering me. When creating a blend for irritability or anxiety associated with PMS, I like to use a blend of nutritive herbs, such as alfalfa and nettles, with nervines such as milky oat tops, lemon balm and passionflower.

Alfalfa, nettles and milky oat tops are rich in vitamins and minerals, which may be helpful in relieving some symptoms of PMS. Supporting the nervous system with herbs such as lemon balm is great for calming the mind and spirit and alleviating anxiety. Passionflower is a fabulous herb for helping to soothe internal self-doubt, mental chatter and mood swings.

INGREDIENTS

3 parts dried milky oat tops

2 parts dried alfalfa

2 parts dried lemon balm

1 part dried passionflower

1 part dried nettle leaf

¼–½ part licorice root

WHAT YOU'LL NEED

Jar, for storage

Kettle

French press or 1-qt (1-L) jar

Strainer

TO MAKE THE HERBAL BLEND

First, decide how much of the tea blend you'd like to make. I use cups for the parts, so I have a large batch that will last me a couple of weeks. Using cups makes about 10½ cups (300 g) of the blend. If using ½ cup for the parts, then it would make about 5¼ cups (150 g) of the blend. If you're looking to make just a couple of cups of infusion or tea, then I suggest using tablespoon measurements, which will give you just over ½ cup (15 g) of blend.

Once you've figured out how much you want to make, start measuring the herbs into a mixing bowl. Get right in there and use your hands to mix the herbs until it comes together into a lovely cohesive blend. Store in a jar until ready to use.

TO MAKE THE INFUSION

Heat up some water in a kettle or pot. Use a ratio of 1 to 2 tablespoons (2 to 4 g) of the herb blend to each 1 cup (240 ml) of boiling water. You can fill the French press or quart jar completely or just make a small amount, it's up to you. Once you've decided how much you'd like to make, place the herb blend into the French press or jar. Once the water has boiled, add it to the vessel with herbs. If using a jar, cover with a lid, and if using a French press, make sure not to press down on the herbs until after they've had time to infuse. Let steep for at least 2 hours or up to 12 hours.

If you want to make a refreshing chilled drink, make it at night and place it in the fridge before bed. The next day you will have a delicious and refreshing infusion! Serve over ice and enjoy.

TO MAKE THE TEA

Follow the instructions above except only let steep for 5 to 20 minutes and serve warm.

PMS SUPPORT TINCTURE

Makes 6–8 oz (180–240 ml)

This recipe offers a number of options. We're all different and experience our cycles differently. Some people may be heavy bleeders or have bad cramping while someone else might be a really light bleeder but have a lot of anxiety. The suggestions below are meant to give you choices depending on your needs. For instance, maybe you have cramping, heavy bleeding and anxiety with palpitations. Then I would recommend cramp bark, yarrow, rose and motherwort.

Learn the plants. Once you have a better understanding of each individual plant, you will then be able to tailor the formula to suit your needs best.

TINCTURE

2 oz (60 ml) fresh milky oat tincture or 6 tbsp (8 g) fresh milky oat tops (see Note)

2 tbsp (3 g) dried raspberry leaf

1 tbsp (11 g) dried burdock root

2 tsp (6 g) dried angelica root

1–2 tbsp (20–40 g) honey (optional)

1 cup (240 ml) vodka or brandy

OPTIONAL ADDITIONS

For Cramping

2 tsp (6 g) dried cramp bark

1 tsp dried ginger pieces

For Heavy Bleeding

1 tsp dried yarrow

1 tsp dried black haw

For Anxiety

2 tsp (2 g) dried skullcap

2 tsp (2 g) dried lemon balm

For Anxiety with Heart Palpitations

2 tsp (2 g) dried motherwort

WHAT YOU'LL NEED

Spice grinder

8-oz (240-ml) jar

Strainer

4 (2-oz [60-ml]) dropper bottles or a jar, for storage

Once you've decided on your herbs, gather them and one by one, measure them out, run them through a spice grinder and then place in an 8-ounce (240-ml) jar. If using honey, you can add it now. Next, pour in the vodka until the jar is filled. Mix it all together and add more alcohol if needed to top off the jar. Then place the cap on and shake. Open the jar back up and check to see if the alcohol level has dropped. If it has, add more to the jar and cover back up.

Label your jar and let sit for 4 weeks. Store in a place where you'll see it often. Shake it every week and taste a drop or two. After 4 weeks, you can strain and bottle into labeled 2-ounce (60-ml) dropper bottles or a jar.

TO USE

Take 1 full dropper (¼ teaspoon) one to three times per day in water or tea, as needed.

Note: This blend will be most effective using fresh milky oat tops. If you aren't able to source them fresh, you can purchase prepared fresh milky oat tincture from an herbal shop and use 2 ounces (60 ml) in this blend. Dried milky oat tops make a lovely infusion, but they don't come close to comparing to the medicinal activity of fresh milky oat tops when making a tincture. You can use an equal amount of dried, just be aware the tincture may not be as effective.

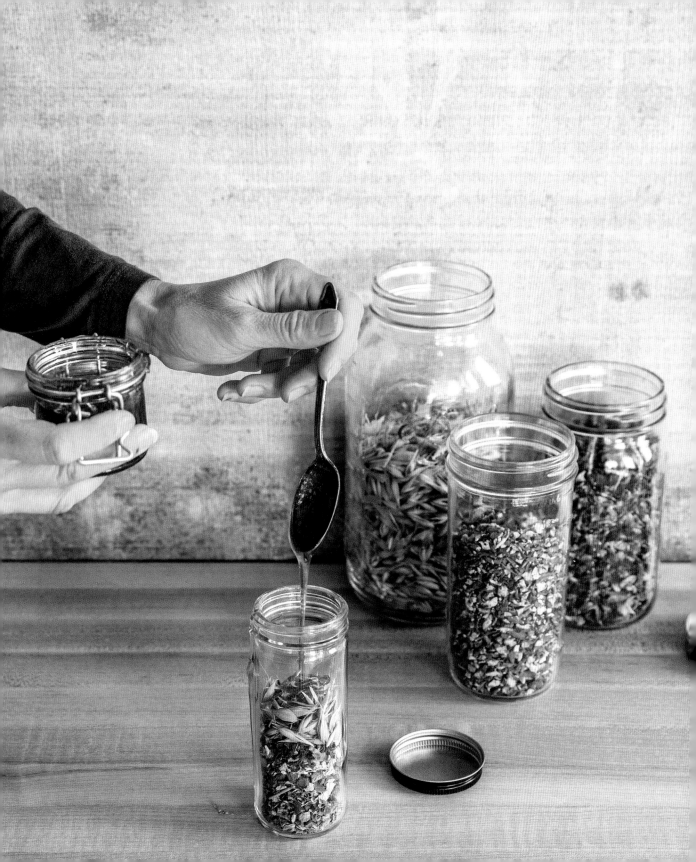

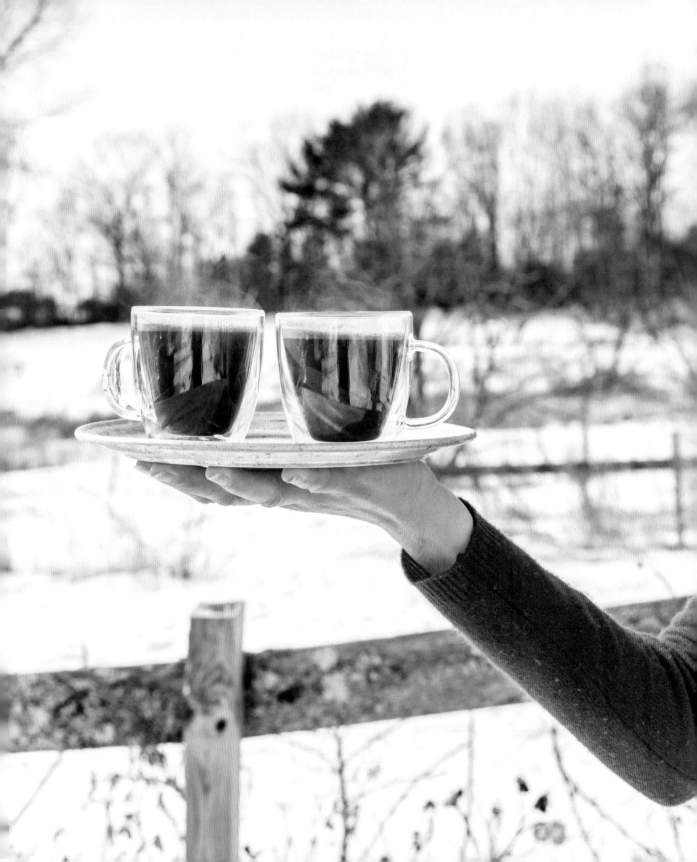

"LET'S GET IT ON (OR NOT)" HOT CHOCOLATE FERTILITY TEA

Pregnancy looks different for everyone, and it's not just a woman and man, or husband and wife. There are so many wonderful situations and scenarios. No matter what your situation, if you're trying to conceive, this is a tasty way to support fertility.

Almost all of us love chocolate, and what a wonderful and sacred way to enjoy a cup, either alone or with someone else that you love and care for.

Makes enough tea blend for
7 cups (1.4 L) of tea

INGREDIENTS

3 tbsp (28 g) raw cacao powder

1 tbsp (9 g) dried shatavari powder

1 tsp dried ashwagandha powder

1 tsp maca powder

½ tsp cinnamon powder

Pinch of nutmeg

Your favorite milk (regular
or plant-based)

Maple syrup or honey to taste

WHAT YOU'LL NEED

Spice grinder

8-oz (240-ml) jar

Small pot

Strainer

Immersion blender or
blender (optional)

When making medicine, holding intent and vision is an important part of the process, making it sacred. As you're gathering your herbs, meditate on why you're making this blend. This is a powerful aspect to making medicine, being clear with intent and putting our energy into it. Hold your reasons for making this medicine close to you while going through the following steps.

Gather your herbs and, using a spice grinder, grind the herbs that are not already in powder form. Place all the powdered herbs in a bowl and use a spoon to mix them all together until nicely blended. If you don't have a grinder, you can just measure out the herbs and mix them together in a bowl. Store in a jar.

When you're ready to make tea, fill your mug with milk a quarter to halfway full. Fill the rest of the mug up with water; you should have about 1 cup (240 ml) of liquid. You could also use all milk if you prefer.

Pour the liquid from the mug into a pot and measure out 2 teaspoons (6 g) of the tea blend. Warm the mixture over medium-high heat. Once it reaches a simmer, lower the heat and let it simmer for 5 to 10 minutes. Then remove it from the heat.

If you'd like, you can strain the mixture, or simply pour it into your mug (you'll want to strain it if you didn't use a grinder). Add some maple syrup to taste for a little sweetness and more milk if you'd like it creamier.

For an extra frothy treat, you can pour it all into a blender or use a handheld immersion blender and blend for 5 to 10 seconds. Enjoy!

PREGNANCY SUPPORT INFUSION

Yield varies

Once you're pregnant it's all about keeping yourself strong and nourished. Pregnancy can be taxing both physically and mentally. So, it's important to make sure you're getting enough vitamins and minerals through supplements, food and herbs. This tea makes a wonderful and supportive addition to your daily health regime. To address specific common issues in pregnancy, add one or more of the listed options to the base tea blend.

INFUSION

2 parts dried nettle leaf

2 parts dried milky oat tops

1 part dried lemon balm

1 part dried alfalfa

½ part dried mint

OPTIONAL ADDITIONS

For Nausea

½–1 part dried ginger pieces

For Water Retention

1 part dried dandelion roots

For Tension and Stress

2 parts dried lemon balm

WHAT YOU'LL NEED

Jar, for storage

Kettle

French press or 1-qt (1-L) jar for tea

Strainer

First, decide how much of the tea blend you'd like to make. I use cups for the parts, which makes 6 to 8 cups (130 to 170 g) of the blend, so I have a large batch that will last me a couple of weeks. If you're looking to make just a couple of cups of infusion or tea, then I suggest using tablespoon measurements, which will give you about ½ cup (11 g) of blend.

Once you've figured out how much you want to make, measure the herbs into a mixing bowl and blend with your hands. You know the drill. Add the herbs to the jar, label it, place the cap on and store it until ready to make the infusion.

When ready to make the infusion, heat some water in a kettle or pot. Take a good handful or two of the herbs, ½ to 1 cup (11 to 22 g) total, and put them in a French press or jar and add the boiling water. If using a jar, cover with a lid, and if using a French press, make sure not to press down on the herbs until after they've had time to infuse. Let sit and infuse for at least 2 hours and up to 12 hours. Sometimes I will make this at nighttime and if it's summer, I will put it in the fridge before going to bed. Then it makes a great iced tea the next day.

Drink every day throughout the day, or as needed.

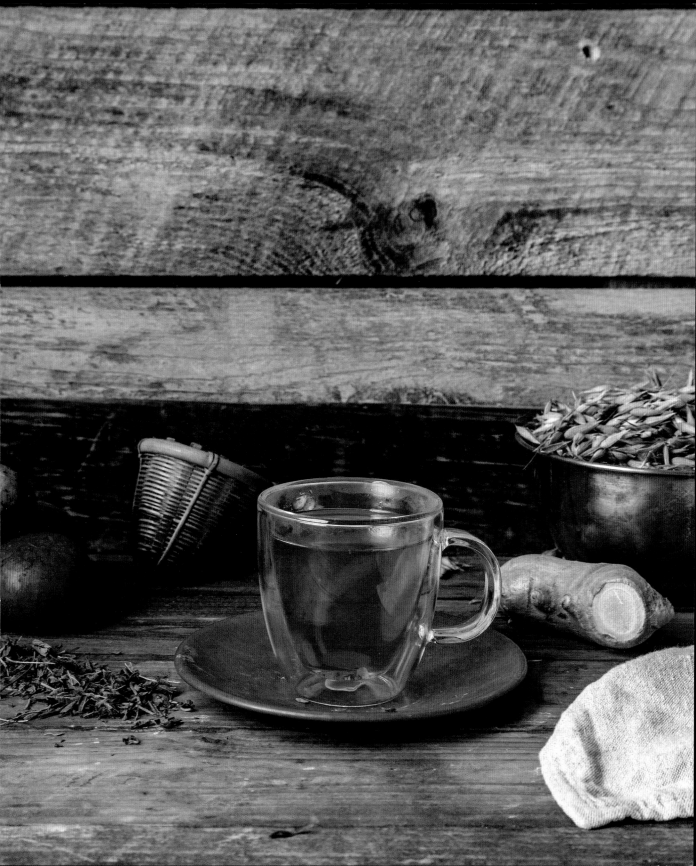

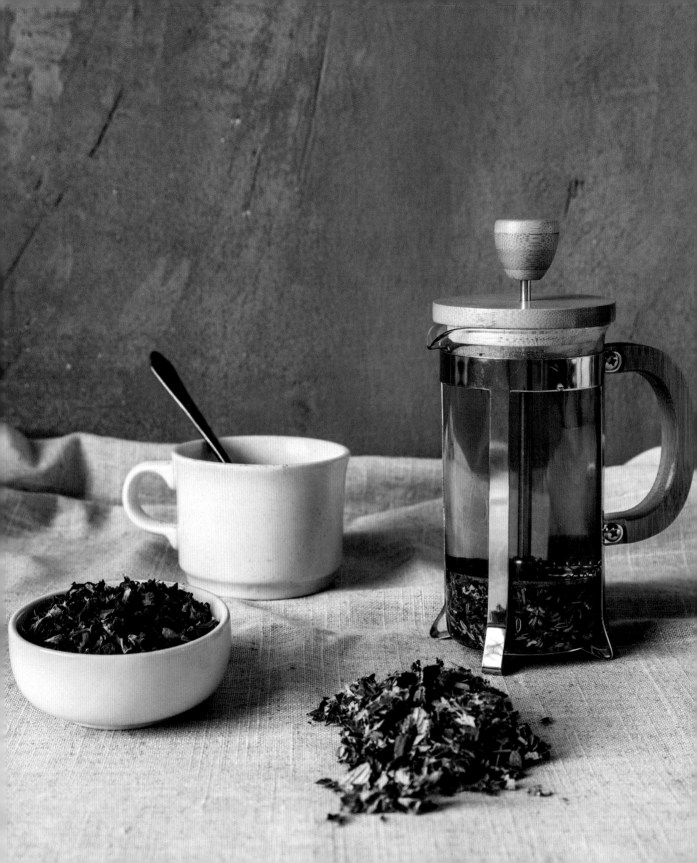

"BABY'S HERE, NOW WHAT?" INFUSION

Makes 14–16 cups (350–400 g)

The weeks and months after a baby is born are an important time for the birth mother to support her body with herbs that nourish and tone the uterus and reproductive system. Your body has just been through a lot, so try to be patient with it, as it can take time for the hormones to balance and for the dust to settle. It's also a time to adjust to the fact that you're a new mom, probably not getting a lot of sleep.

Raspberry leaf and lady's mantle are both uterine tonics and can help tone and restore the uterus. They can also be helpful in lessening any excessive postpartum bleeding. Nettles, milky oat tops and raspberry leaf are nutritive herbs that are restorative, helping to build back your reserves; lemon balm and milky oat tops support your nervous system as well. You'll see this recipe offers choices to tailor it to your specific needs, so feel free to add the herbs you need to the base recipe. This recipe makes a big batch, so you can have plenty on hand to support your healing journey in the weeks and months to come. This would also make a fantastic gift to a new mom, packed in a large jar with ribbon.

INFUSION

4 cups (116 g) dried nettle

4 cups (80 g) dried milky oat tops

2 cups (40 g) dried raspberry leaf

2 cups (58 g) dried lemon balm

2 cup (58 g) dried lady's mantle

OPTIONAL ADDITIONS

To Support Milk Production

1 cup (104 g) dried fennel seeds

For Heavy Bleeding

2 cups (40 g) dried yarrow leaf and flower

2 cups (19 g) dried shepherd's purse

For Postpartum Depression

2 cups (20 g) dried rose petals

1 cup (20 g) dried tulsi

WHAT YOU'LL NEED

2 (½-gal [2-L]) jars or 1 (1-gal [4-L]) jar

32-oz (900-g) jar or French press

Kettle

Strainer

As you begin to gather your herbs, a nice practice is to hold your intentions for why you're making this blend. Is it to help balance hormones and excess bleeding? Is it to help restore energy and uplift your mood and spirit? Whatever your intention, hold it throughout the infusion-making process.

Gather all your herbs and measure them into a bowl. Still holding your intention, gently blend all the herbs together using your hands. Once well blended, store in either two ½-gallon (2-L) jars or one 1-gallon (4-L) jar.

When ready to make the infusion, place ½ to 1 cup (12 to 25 g) of herb blend into either a jar or a French press. Bring 4 cups (960 ml) of water to a boil in a pot or kettle, and pour it over the herbs. If using a jar, cover with a lid, and if using a French press, make sure not to press down on the herbs until after they've had time to infuse. Let it steep for at least 1 hour and up to 12 hours

I like to make the infusion in the morning and start enjoying it by midday, or make it at night so it's ready to go in the morning. You can enjoy it at room temperature or for something warmer, strain and warm the tea back up in a pan over low heat for 5 minutes or until you've reached the desired temperature. If you want it chilled, just put it in the fridge before bed for a tasty iced tea the next day.

HEALING SUPPORT TINCTURE + INFUSION FOR A MISCARRIAGE OR ABORTION

Makes 6–8 oz (180–240 ml) tincture,
⅓ cup (22 g) loose-leaf tea blend

This is a formula to have on hand if you plan to have an abortion or have a history of miscarriages. Since this tincture takes a few weeks, I suggest making it once you find out you're pregnant. If you decide to have an abortion or end up with a miscarriage, this tincture will be there, ready for when you need it. If you need something faster, you can make the infusion; it won't be as powerful as the tincture, but may still be effective.

In times of need, the herbs are there for us. Our bodies need much love and support during abortions and miscarriages, and herbs such as lady's mantle, raspberry leaf and yarrow can be very supportive. Lady's mantle is astringent and a fabulous uterine tonic that can help with excessive bleeding. Raspberry leaf is a wonderful nutritive and uterine tonic. It can help with tone and restore the uterus, and it can help lessen the amount of bleeding and possibly pain. Yarrow is astringent and antispasmodic, making it helpful for any painful cramping.

Hopefully, you're able to take time for yourself to do what you need to do before jumping back into the full swing of life.

INGREDIENTS

2 tbsp (2 g) dried lady's mantle

2 tbsp (2 g) dried raspberry leaf

1 tbsp (1 g) dried motherwort

1 tbsp (11 g) dried burdock

1 tsp dried yarrow

About 1 cup (240 ml) vodka
(for tincture)

WHAT YOU'LL NEED

Spice grinder

8-oz (240-ml) jar (for tincture) or
1-qt (1-L) jar or 32-oz (900-g)
French press (for infusion)

Strainer

4 (2-oz [60-ml]) dropper bottles
or a jar, for storage
(for tincture)

Kettle

TO MAKE THE TINCTURE

Gather your herbs. One by one measure them out and run them through your grinder, then place into an 8-ounce (240-ml) jar. If you don't have a grinder, you can just measure out the herbs and place directly into the jar.

Next, pour in the vodka until the jar is filled. Mix it all together and add more alcohol if needed, then place the cap on and shake. Open the jar back up and check to see if the alcohol level has dropped. If it has, add more to the jar and cover back up.

Label your jar and let sit for 4 weeks. Store in a place where you'll see it often. Shake it every week and taste a drop or two. After 4 weeks, strain and bottle in labeled 2-ounce (60-ml) dropper bottles or a jar.

TO USE THE TINCTURE

Take 1 full dropper (¼ teaspoon) one to three times a day for a month or until your cycle returns to normal.

TO MAKE THE INFUSION

Combine the herbs in a bowl with your hands, then add them to a 1-quart (1-L) jar or 32-ounce (900-g) French press. Pour boiling water over the herbs to fill the jar or French press. Let it infuse for at least 2 hours and up to 12 hours.

TO USE THE INFUSION

Drink 1 to 2 cups (240 to 480 ml) daily until your cycle returns to normal. Store in the fridge for up to 1 day.

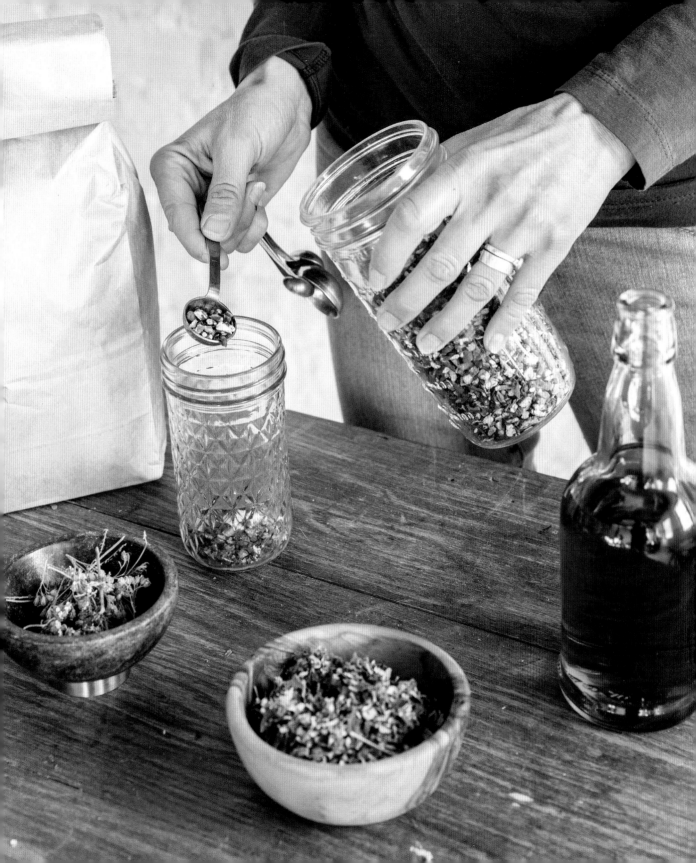

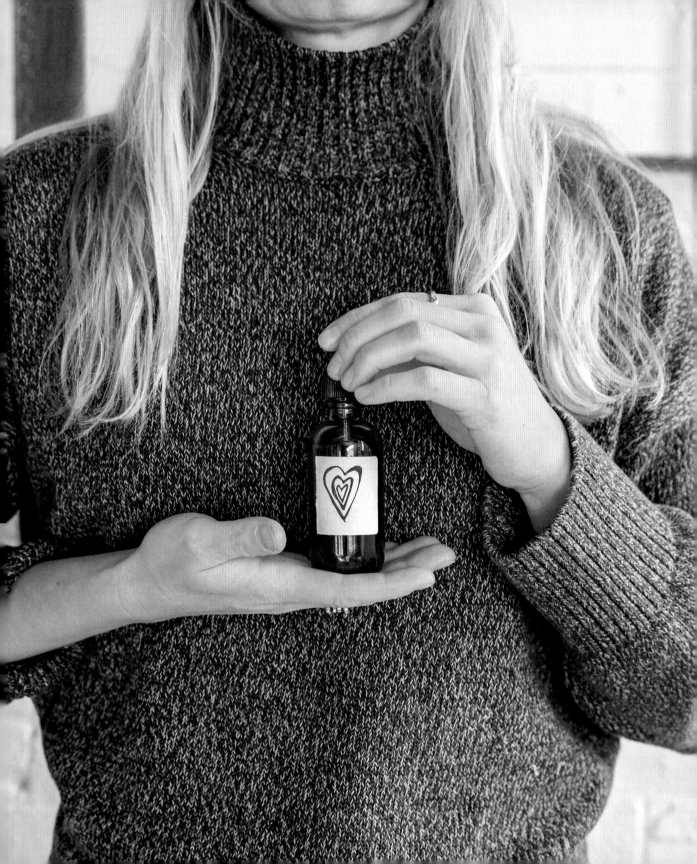

EMOTIONAL WELL-BEING TINCTURE + TEA FOR A MISCARRIAGE OR ABORTION

Makes 6–8 oz (180–240 ml) tincture, roughly ¾ cup (150 g) loose-leaf tea

Whether it's a miscarriage or the decision to have an abortion, the energetic and emotional well-being needs support. This formula has nervines and sedatives in it such as hops, California poppy and lemon balm. These herbs can help with the emotional aspects of having an abortion or a miscarriage, such as anxiety, sleeplessness and physical and emotional pain.

This blend can be used in conjunction with the Healing Support Tincture + Infusion for a Miscarriage or Abortion (page 96) or on its own. This can be made into a tincture or a tea. The formula benefits from the addition of flower essence support, so I've included a few options.

When making medicine, holding intent and vision is an important part of the process, especially with this blend for healing the emotional and the physical. As you're gathering your herbs, meditate on why you're making this tincture, whether it's for yourself, a family member or a friend in need. Holding your reasons for making this medicine close to you while going through the following steps is a powerful part of the medicine making.

TINCTURE + TEA

3 tbsp (5 g) dried lemon balm

2 tbsp (6 g) dried skullcap

2 tbsp (6 g) dried California poppy, leaf, flower and root

1 tbsp (1 g) dried rose petals

1 tbsp (1 g) dried hops

1–2 tbsp (20–40 g) honey (optional)

About 1 cup (240 ml) vodka or brandy (for tincture)

OPTIONAL FLOWER ESSENCE ADDITIONS

Bleeding heart—helps us let go

Borage—helps soothe grief of a miscarriage or an abortion

WHAT YOU'LL NEED

Spice grinder

8-oz (240-ml) jar

Strainer

4 (2-oz [60-ml]) dropper bottles or a jar, for storage

Kettle

TO MAKE THE TINCTURE

Gather your herbs and one by one measure them out and run them through a spice grinder, then place into the 8-ounce (240-ml) jar. If you don't have a grinder, you can just measure out the herbs and place directly into the jar. If using honey, you can add it now. Next, pour in the vodka until the jar is filled. Mix it together and add more vodka if needed to top off the jar. Then place the cap on and shake. Open the jar back up and check to see if the alcohol level has dropped. If it has, add more to the jar and cover back up.

Label your jar and let sit for 4 weeks. Store in a place where you'll see it often. Shake it every week and taste a drop or two. After 4 weeks, strain into a bowl or jar.

At this time, if using flower essences, you can add 5 drops of each one you decide to use. Gently stir the flower essence in. Bottle in labeled 2-ounce (60-ml) dropper bottles or a jar.

TO USE THE TINCTURE

Take 1 to 2 full droppers (¼ to ½ teaspoon) one to three times a day until you feel your nervous system, emotional heart and sleep patterns return to where you would like.

TO MAKE THE TEA

Blend the dry herbs in the jar. Use 2 teaspoons (2 g) of herb blend per 1 cup (240 ml) of boiling water. Let steep for 10 to 15 minutes, then strain into a cup. You can add 1 or 2 drops of one or both of the flower essences.

TO USE THE TEA

Drink 1 to 3 cups (240 to 720 ml) a day as needed.

IRON MAIDEN SYRUP

Makes 24 oz (710 ml)

I've always wanted to have a product called Iron Maiden in my herb shop, but in order for syrups to be shelf stable they need to be either high in sugar or alcohol or made with glycerin—yuck. So, I've never offered it. This syrup will not be indefinitely shelf stable, but it will last for 2 months when stored in the refrigerator. I find this recipe to be most powerful if it's made by the person who needs it and/or by someone caring for that person. A great deal of the goodness comes from cooking and simmering the plants in the water.

Made with herbs such as nettles, ashwagandha and alfalfa, this is a great herbal supplement to help build up stores of iron, minerals and vitamins as well as vitality and strength. All of them are nutritive, making them useful for building us up from depletion. Nettles are packed with minerals and vitamins. As a blood-building herb, it is beneficial for iron-deficient anemia and fatigue. Ashwagandha is rich in iron, making it another great herb for anemia. Additionally, alfalfa is useful for helping restock our stores of folate.

INGREDIENTS

½ cup (31 g) dried nettle

⅓ cup (6 g) dried raspberry leaf

2 tbsp (22 g) dried dandelion root

2 tbsp (22 g) dried burdock root

⅓ cup (12 g) dried alfalfa

2 tbsp (10 g) dried astragalus

2 tbsp (7 g) dried yellow dock root

2 tbsp (16 g) dried ashwagandha

2 qt (2 L) water

½–1 cup (120–240 ml) maple syrup or (160–320 g) honey

3 tbsp (60 g) molasses (preferably organic blackstrap)

1 tbsp (5 g) rose hip powder

¼ cup (60 ml) brandy (optional)

WHAT YOU'LL NEED

3-qt (3-L) pot

Strainer

32-oz (946-ml) jar, for storage

Gather all the herbs and place them in a 3-quart (3-L) pot. Add the water to the pot, cover and let the water and herbs infuse at room temperature for 2 to 4 hours.

Next, set the pot over high heat. Bring to a boil and then reduce to a low simmer. The goal is to reduce the liquid down to 2 cups (480 ml), which usually takes 2 or more hours. Once you've got it down to about 2 cups (480 ml), remove from the heat and strain into the 32-ounce (946-ml) jar. If your liquid ends up being less than 2 cups (480 ml), that's fine, just add some water back to your reduced liquid until it measures 2 cups (480 ml).

Now it's time to add the maple syrup or honey to the jar. I prefer maple syrup because it's just so friggin' good, but honey is amazing as well. Stir it in well. Next, add the molasses, rose hip powder and brandy (if using). Mix well.

Label the jar and store it in the fridge for up to 2 months.

TO USE
Take 1 tablespoon (15 ml), or, my preferred method, sip a small amount straight from the jar, once a day as needed.

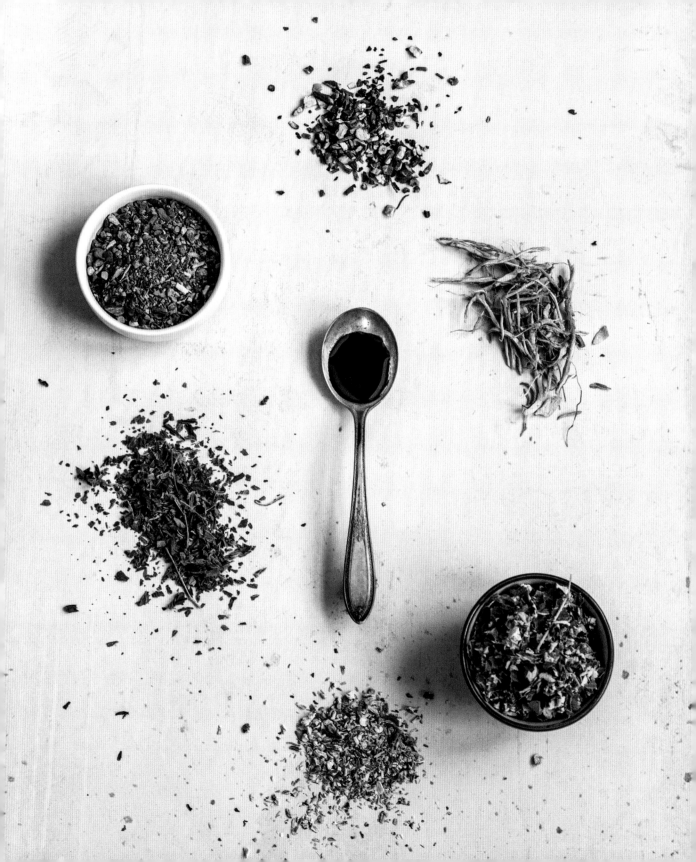

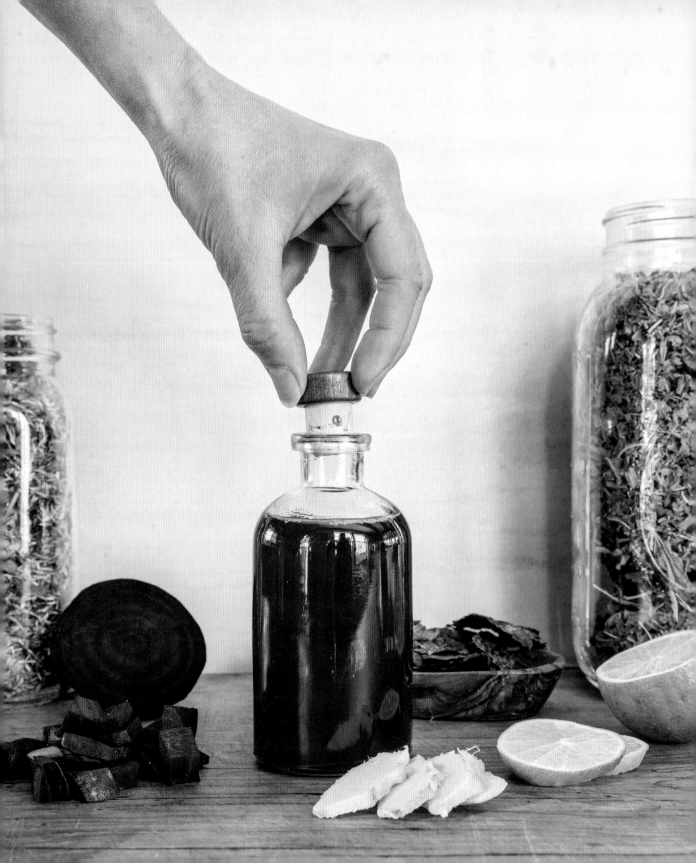

RESTORATIVE VINEGAR

Makes 32 oz (1 L)

Here at the farm I grow almost all of the herbs and vegetables that go into this blend. Made with nutrient-rich beets, nettles, alfalfa and kelp, this blend is not only delicious, but it's also a gorgeous deep purple/pink color. This tonic is a great way to add more nutrient-dense herbs and vegetables to your daily health routine, and it makes a wonderful blend for women of all ages and phases in their lives. I like to use this blend for helping build and restore vitality in the body that can often be depleted after menstruation or giving birth and with aging.

I love working with herbal vinegar because it's a food. I use this blend on roasted vegetables, salads, grains and soups. You can also add it to still or sparkling water and enjoy as a tasty, revitalizing shrub with a touch of honey and a squeeze of lime.

INGREDIENTS

1–2 cups (190–380 g) grated or roughly chopped fresh beets

2 tbsp (18 g) grated fresh ginger

1 cup (54 g) fresh nettles

½ cup (11 g) dried red clover blossom and leaves

¾ cup (18 g) dried milky oat tops

1 cup (23 g) dried alfalfa

¾ cup (15 g) dried raspberry leaf

2 tbsp (20 g) dried kelp

½–1½ cups (160–480 g) honey (optional)

1 tbsp (15 ml) freshly squeezed lime juice

4 cups (960 ml) raw apple cider vinegar

WHAT YOU'LL NEED

1-qt (1-L) jar with BPA-free plastic lid or cheesecloth and a metal lid

Strainer

Jars or bottles, for storage

Place the beets and ginger in a 1-quart (1-L) jar. Then begin measuring and adding all the herbs to the jar. If using honey, add it now, along with the lime juice. Fill the jar with the apple cider vinegar. You can start with ½ cup (160 g) honey, then taste the vinegar and see if you'd like to add more. Cover the jar with either a plastic lid or cheesecloth under the metal lid.

Label the jar and let sit for 4 to 6 weeks in a dark spot out of direct heat, but where you'll see it often. Throughout the weeks, check on the vinegar level in the jar, topping it off with more vinegar if needed.

After 4 to 6 weeks, strain into clean labeled jars or bottles for storage. Enjoy liberally with foods, dressings, sauces or on its own as a drink. I tend to do 1 tablespoon (15 ml) in 1 cup (240 ml) of water. If you wanted to take it more concentrated, you could do a 1-to-1 ratio of vinegar to water.

PERIMENOPAUSE + MENOPAUSE SUPPORT TINCTURE

Makes 6–8 oz (180–240 ml)

There is power that comes from this inner shift in a woman's life. We've turned another corner and there is so much waiting for us in the years ahead. But in order to harness that power from within, we need to support and balance our body and hormones.

As our ovaries retire from making estrogen, symptoms associated with low estrogen may arise and they can be frustrating. Herbs such as vitex, alfalfa and licorice root can help balance and nourish our reproductive and endocrine systems. Vitex has long been revered as an ally to women in relieving night sweats, hot flashes, anxiety and irritability. I like to use motherwort to help with irritability, anxiety and heart palpitations, along with hot flashes and night sweats. Licorice root is a great herb that synergistically brings the formula together while playing a role in lessening the symptoms of night sweats and hot flashes.

INGREDIENTS

2 tbsp (13 g) dried chaste tree berries

2 tbsp (6 g) dried motherwort

1 tbsp (10 g) dried dandelion root

1 tbsp (3 g) dried alfalfa

1 tsp dried licorice root (see Note)

1 tsp cinnamon chips

About 1 cup (240 ml) vodka or brandy

WHAT YOU'LL NEED

Spice grinder

8-oz (240-ml) jar

Strainer

4 (2-oz [60-ml]) dropper bottles or jar, for storage

As you begin to gather your herbs, a nice practice is to hold your intentions for why you're making this blend. Is it to help balance hormones, reduce anxiety or help restore energy? Whatever your intention, hold it throughout the tincture-making process.

Gather your herbs and one by one measure them out and run them through a spice grinder, then place them into an 8-ounce (240-ml) jar. If you don't have a grinder, you can just measure out the herbs and place directly into the jar. Next, pour in the vodka until the jar is filled. Stir the herbs around in the jar and add more vodka if needed to top off the jar. Then place the cap on and shake. Open the jar back up and check to see if the alcohol level has dropped. If it has, add more to the jar and cover back up.

Label your jar and let sit for 4 weeks. Store in a place where you'll see it often. Shake it every week and taste a drop or two. After 4 weeks, strain and bottle in labeled 2-oz (60-ml) dropper bottles or a jar.

TO USE

Take 1 full dropper (¼ teaspoon) one to three times daily, in water or tea, as needed.

Note: Omit licorice root from the formula if you have hypertension, congestive heart failure, edema, hyperkalemia or kidney disease. Omit it if you are taking digoxin, MAOIs, SSRIs, diuretics, antihypertensives or anticoagulants.

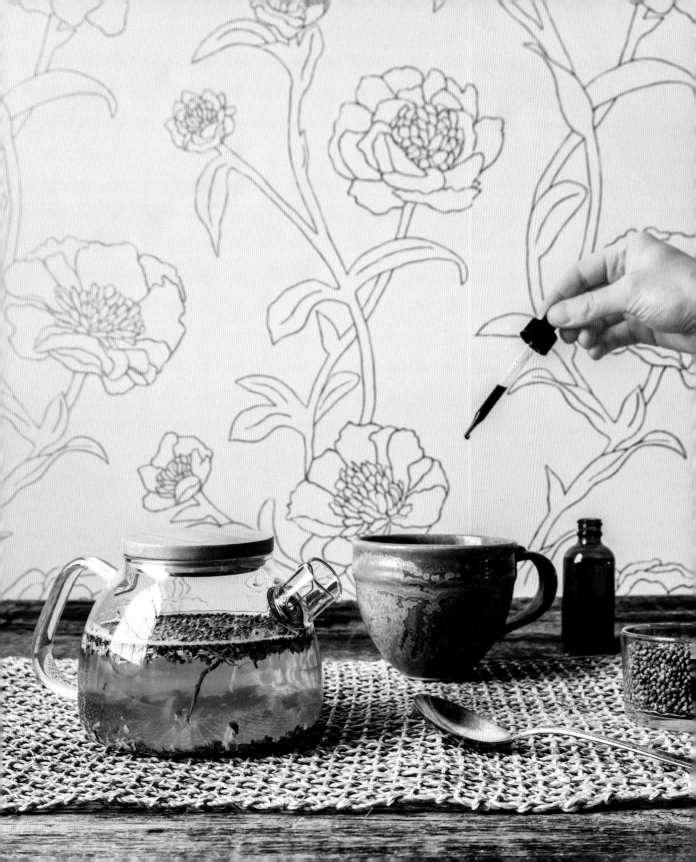

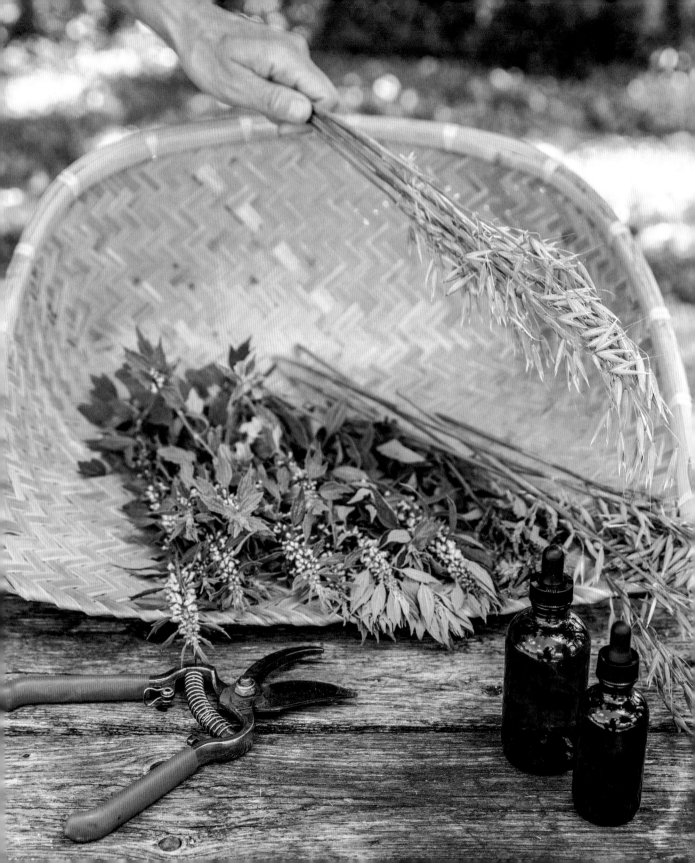

EMOTIONAL SUPPORT TINCTURE FOR PERIMENOPAUSE + MENOPAUSE

Makes 6–8 oz (180–240 ml)

It's important to recognize the need for emotional support in all phases of our lives. As our bodies change and age, it can be incredibly frustrating, especially as we start to deal with perimenopause and menopause. We go from having somewhat predictable hormone cycles to a lot of unpredictability, and with it can come anxiety, nervous stress, insomnia and irritability.

This blend is made with some herbs such as milky oat tops, rose and shatavari that will nurture the nervous, endocrine and reproductive systems. Milky oat tops are deeply nourishing to the endocrine system and supportive to the reproductive and nervous systems. It can help with anxiety, nervous exhaustion, agitation and overreaction. I have always found rose to be gentle and supportive to the cardiovascular, nervous and reproductive systems, helping with irritability and anxiety. Shatavari is likewise supportive of the endocrine and reproductive systems and can help with fatigue and hormonal support.

INGREDIENTS

2 oz (60 ml) fresh milky oat tincture or 6 tbsp (8 g) fresh milky oat tops (see Note)

2 tbsp (17 g) dried shatavari

1 tbsp (4 g) dried motherwort

1 tbsp (1 g) dried rose petals

1 tsp dried blue vervain

1–2 tbsp (20–40 g) honey (optional)

About 1 cup (240 ml) vodka or brandy

WHAT YOU'LL NEED

Spice grinder

8-oz (240-ml) jar

Strainer

4 (2-oz [60-ml]) dropper bottles or a jar, for storage

When making medicine, holding intent and vision is an important part of the process, especially with this blend for healing the emotional heart. As you're gathering your herbs, meditate on why you're making this tincture, whether it's for yourself, a family member or a friend in need. Hold your reasons for making this medicine close to you while going through the following steps.

Gather your herbs and one by one measure them out, run them through a spice grinder and then place in an 8-ounce (240-ml) jar. If you don't have a grinder, you can just measure out the herbs and place directly into the jar. If using honey, you can add it now. Next, pour in the vodka until the jar is filled. Mix it together and add more vodka if needed to top off the jar. Then place the cap on and shake. Open the jar back up and check to see if the alcohol level has dropped. If it has, add more to the jar and cover back up.

Label the jar and let sit for 4 weeks. Store in a place where you'll see it often. Shake it every week and taste a drop or two. After 4 weeks, strain and bottle in labeled 2-ounce (60-ml) dropper bottles or a jar.

TO USE

Take 1 full dropper (¼ teaspoon) in water or tea one to three times a day as needed.

Note: This blend will be most effective using fresh milky oat tops. If you aren't able to source them fresh, you can purchase prepared fresh milky oat tincture from an herbal shop and use 2 ounces (60 ml) in this blend. Dried milky oat tops make a lovely infusion, but they don't come close to comparing to the medicinal activity of fresh milky oat tops when making a tincture. You can use an equal amount of dried, just be aware the tincture may not be as effective.

SLEEP SUPPORT TINCTURE FOR PERIMENOPAUSE + MENOPAUSE

Makes 6–8 oz (180–240 ml)

One of the many symptoms that happens with hormonal shifts can be sleep issues, especially sleep issues where you fall asleep but then wake up and can't get back to sleep. So frustrating! Herbs such as passionflower, hops and motherwort can be helpful during these times.

Passionflower is a beautiful plant and a wonderful nervine and mild sedative. It's a great plant to have close by if you're like me and have trouble shutting down your thoughts at night. It helps quiet the mind and can be especially useful if you wake in the middle of the night and can't get back to sleep. Hops, another beauty, is an aromatic bitter, sedative and anxiolytic. I use it for anxiety and insomnia, and because it's a digestive it can be helpful for stress and sleep disturbances related to digestion. Motherwort is also a fabulous nervine and cardiotonic. It can be helpful if you are having issues waking in the night with heart palpitations. I also like it to help balance unpredictable emotions due to hormones, helping to calm the nerves, relieve stress and encourage sleep.

INGREDIENTS

1 tbsp (4 g) dried passionflower

1 tbsp (1 g) dried hops

2 tsp (2 g) dried motherwort

2 tsp (2 g) dried California poppy, leaf, flower and roots

1 tsp dried chaste tree berry

About 1 cup (240 ml) vodka or brandy

WHAT YOU'LL NEED

Spice grinder

8-oz (240-ml) jar

Strainer

4 (2-oz [60-ml]) dropper bottles or a jar, for storage

Gather your herbs and one by one measure them out, run them through a spice grinder and then place in an 8-ounce (240-ml) jar. If you don't have a grinder, you can just measure out the herbs and place directly into the jar. Next, pour in the vodka until the jar is filled. Mix it all together and add more vodka if needed to top off the jar. Then place the cap on and shake. Open the jar back up and check to see if the alcohol level has dropped. If it has, add more to the jar and cover back up.

Label the jar and let sit for 4 weeks. Store in a place where you'll see it often. Shake it every week and taste a drop or two. After 4 weeks, strain and bottle in labeled 2-ounce (60-ml) dropper bottles or a jar.

TO USE

Take 1 full dropper (¼ teaspoon) after dinner and then again before bed. I also suggest keeping a bottle on your nightstand so that if you wake in the night you can easily take a dropperful to help you get back to sleep.

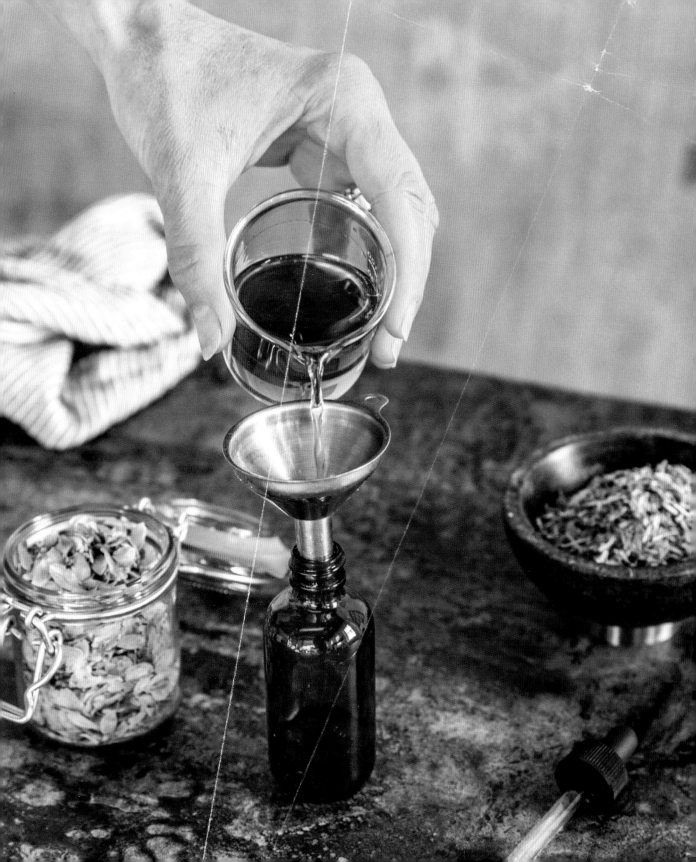

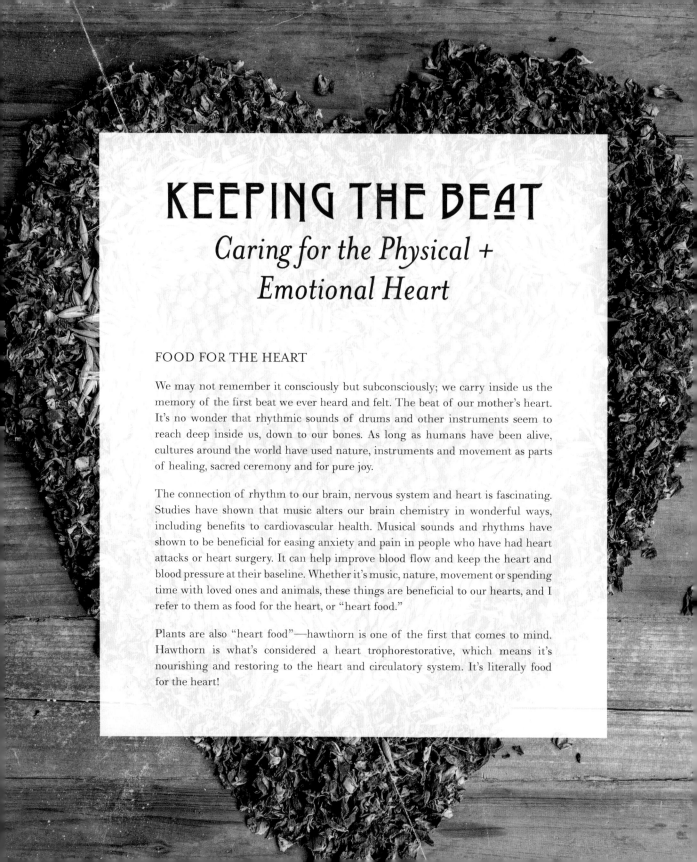

KEEPING THE BEAT
Caring for the Physical +
Emotional Heart

FOOD FOR THE HEART

We may not remember it consciously but subconsciously; we carry inside us the memory of the first beat we ever heard and felt. The beat of our mother's heart. It's no wonder that rhythmic sounds of drums and other instruments seem to reach deep inside us, down to our bones. As long as humans have been alive, cultures around the world have used nature, instruments and movement as parts of healing, sacred ceremony and for pure joy.

The connection of rhythm to our brain, nervous system and heart is fascinating. Studies have shown that music alters our brain chemistry in wonderful ways, including benefits to cardiovascular health. Musical sounds and rhythms have shown to be beneficial for easing anxiety and pain in people who have had heart attacks or heart surgery. It can help improve blood flow and keep the heart and blood pressure at their baseline. Whether it's music, nature, movement or spending time with loved ones and animals, these things are beneficial to our hearts, and I refer to them as food for the heart, or "heart food."

Plants are also "heart food"—hawthorn is one of the first that comes to mind. Hawthorn is what's considered a heart trophorestorative, which means it's nourishing and restoring to the heart and circulatory system. It's literally food for the heart!

THE EMOTIONAL HEART

Our hearts are amazing, supplying our entire body all day long with blood and oxygen. But this brilliant muscle is more than just a pump for moving blood. It carries our emotions and energetics, too.

Unfortunately, we exist in an overwhelming and demanding society, a society that doesn't always honor or even recognize the emotional heart and the importance of feeding it. Yet we live in a day and age when daily anxiety and stress keep our bodies in a constant flight-or-fright state, whether it's from minor daily worries and challenges or bigger picture social issues that affect our communities and the world. "Fight or flight" is a physical reaction caused by the adrenaline hormone, but it is usually set off because of an emotion we're having. When we go into fight or flight, our heart is one of the organs that is affected, and you can feel it pounding in your chest. These constant day-to-day stressors add up and can lead to chronic anxiety, heart attacks, even high blood pressure, angina and overall weakened cardiovascular health.

When we start to ignore the emotional heart, we can grow bitter, distant, frustrated and desensitized. A broken heart is a great example of the physical and emotional heart connection. Most all of us have experienced a broken heart. We feel hurt, sad and vulnerable, but we also during this time might physically feel pain within our hearts as well, or we might start having anxiety with heart palpitations. A broken heart may make us rigid and walled off from others, which can also manifest as stiffness and rigidity within the heart muscle itself.

Have you ever said, "I'm so stressed I'm going to give myself a heart attack"? We know there are a handful of factors involved when it comes to heart disease and heart attacks, and our lifestyle is one of them. This includes our stress levels, emotional and mental health, eating habits, exercise habits and consumption of alcohol, drugs and cigarettes, as well as genetics.

It's normal for people to not intuitively make the connection between the physical and emotional heart, but once the connection is made, it becomes easier to understand and want to address shifts within. There are plenty of statistics out there showing people live happy, longer lives or recover quicker from surgeries and illnesses if they have a pet, some sort of spiritual practice or a loving support group. It's because all this goodness feeds the heart.

I do believe there are instances where not addressing emotions and past or present trauma can play a role in certain health issues, and they can especially play a role in the healing process. However, I want to be clear: Ignoring our emotions doesn't always result in manifesting into a physical ailment or disease. Clearly, there are a lot of reasons to start reducing our stress levels and supporting heart health. Understanding how the heart works and how these diseases manifest in the first place is a step toward prevention. The more we know and understand, the better chances we have of making lasting beneficial changes that will support not only our cardiovascular system but also our body as a whole.

When I'm formulating for the heart, I often take into consideration the emotional heart as well, because it's all connected.

LET'S GET PHYSICAL

The cardiovascular system is made up of our heart, blood vessels and blood. Its role is to deliver nutrients and oxygen to all cells in the body and remove waste, such as carbon dioxide, from the body. Amazing, I know.

An adult has about 11 pints (5.3 L) of blood, making up one-twelfth of our body weight. Blood is responsible for delivering oxygen, nutrients and hormones. Obviously, we think of the blood when we think about supporting the cardiovascular system, but it's important to also support the blood in herbal formulas that address other aspects of the body. Keeping in mind how everything is connected, the blood literally reaches all aspects of the body through our arteries, veins and capillaries. This can be a great visual for connecting all the different systems in the body, like a great river with thousands of streams and brooks branching out from its source.

There are a number of factors that can weaken the heart. We've mentioned how lifestyle plays a big role. If we're eating foods rich in saturated fats, sugars and processed foods, this can lead to the buildup of plaque in the arteries, referred to as atherosclerosis. When plaque builds up in the arteries, it narrows the passageways for oxygen-rich blood to flow, making it more challenging for the rest of the body to receive the proper oxygen and blood it needs to function well. This includes the heart. The heart also needs to work harder to pump the blood through those narrow passageways. Blocked arteries can lead to blood clots and heart attacks, which is the leading cause of death in the United States.

Everything is connected and herbs don't just work on one specific system, because our systems don't work in an isolated way. They work together. There are some great herbs like hawthorn that can help support the cardiovascular system, often as a whole, through building strength within the entire system and beyond while also offering nourishment.

Herbs can offer a lot in the way of preventive care, but they can also be very supportive once disease patterns are present. When creating herbal blends, always meditate on the intention of the formula, and in this case, it would be for the heart. No matter what the situation, I always include herbs that are nourishing and strengthening to the heart, herbal nervines, adaptogens and herbs that are supportive for circulation and potentially diuretics.

I want to stress the importance of working with a health practitioner when it comes to serious heart conditions and any type of medications. This book is all about creating general formulas, when truly we all would benefit from formulas specifically designed for our unique situation. So, if you have heart disease and are currently on medication, please consult with your practitioner and work with a clinical herbalist who is trained in working with heart disease.

HEART HEALTH AND GENETICS

This entire chapter is all about things that we can do to support and take preventive action for cardiovascular health. It's important to understand that sometimes we may have a genetic predisposition because our families have a long history of high blood pressure and heart attacks. While family history and genetics play a role, it's important not to let that history dictate ours as well.

The concern and fear are real, I know. There is a long family history of heart disease on my father's side, with some of those heart attacks resulting in deaths. Thankfully, this was not the case for my father. He survived a major heart attack. Although he had to undergo a massive quintuple bypass heart surgery, it saved his life. That was eighteen years ago.

For a long time, I too was afraid that I would have a heart attack, but here's the thing: We have a lot of control over our heart health; it's not all dictated by genes. We can do our best to support both the physical and the emotional heart through our diets, exercise, lifestyle and, of course, herbs!

My dad is still alive and doing very well. He's done a lot of work over the years in supporting both his physical and his emotional heart. He eats better, exercises regularly and did a lot of work on reducing stress and adding more heart food into his life. He's let a lot of things go and has addressed his own emotional heart and fears of his genetic history. He does take medication, but I truly believe he's in such good health because of all the changes he's made as well. If he were just taking medication and doing none of the other work, I don't think he'd be as healthy as he is.

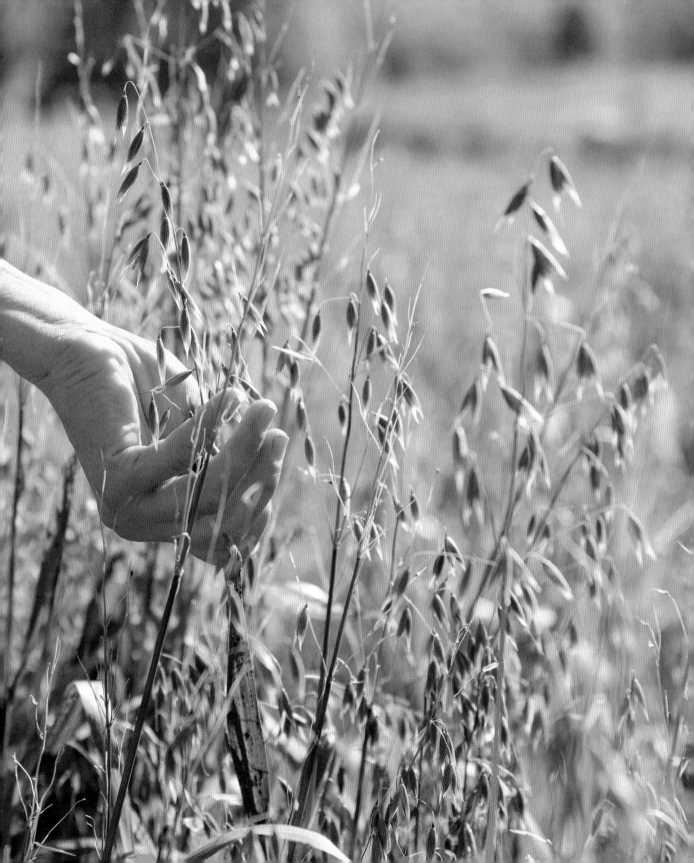

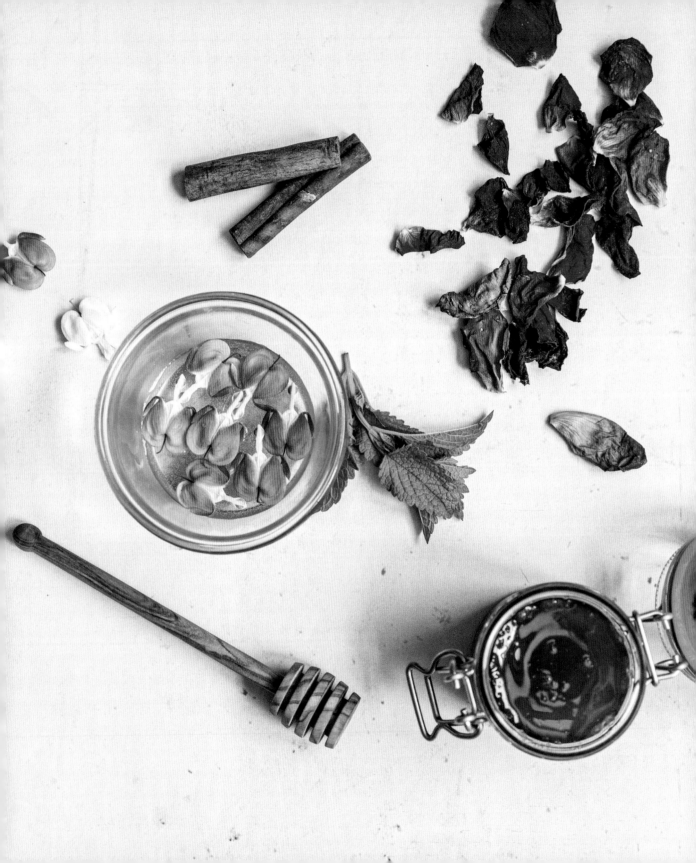

MY BLEEDING HEART CORDIAL

Makes 6–8 oz (180–240 ml)

There are so many ways our hearts can be hurt, and I believe it's important that we allow ourselves to feel and process. I also believe it's important to support ourselves through the process. This tasty cordial is made with herbs such as rose, linden and hawthorn that support the heart and nervous system both physically and energetically.

Rose is a wonderful nervine and cardiotonic. I love using it for support when moving through heartache, grief and anxiety. Rose uplifts the heart. Linden is an antidepressant, nervine and cardiotonic, making it great for helping with anxiety, depression and sleep. Hawthorn is a cardio trophorestorative, nervine and vasodilator. I use hawthorn in all my heart formulas to help support the heart and circulatory system, along with using it to help with anxiety, palpitations, aching heart, grief and stagnant depression. Flower essences also make a nice addition to this cordial, so I've included some options for those as well.

CORDIAL

2 tbsp (3 g) dried rose petals

1 tbsp (13 g) dried hawthorn berries

1 tbsp (2 g) dried milky oat tops

2 tsp (3 g) dried linden

2 tsp (1 g) dried lemon balm

1 tsp dried cinnamon chips

2 tbsp (40 g) honey

About 1 cup (240 ml) brandy

OPTIONAL FLOWER ESSENCE ADDITIONS

Bleeding heart—helps us process and accept loss, such as the end of a relationship or the death of a loved one, and helps support a broken heart

Borage—uplifts the heart and creates courage to face challenges

Forget-me-not—helps us stay connected and linked to those who have passed to the spirit world

Dandelion—helps release grief and pain caused by our emotions that's become stuck in our body

WHAT YOU'LL NEED

8-oz (240-ml) jar

Strainer

4 (2-oz [60-ml]) dropper bottles or a jar, for storage

When making medicine, holding intent and vision is an important part of the process, especially with this blend for healing the emotional heart. As you're gathering your herbs, meditate on why you're making this tincture, whether it's for yourself, a family member or a friend in need. Hold your reasons for making this medicine close to you while going through the following steps.

Gather your herbs and start measuring out all the herbs into the jar. Next, add the honey and then the brandy. Cover and shake, shake, shake.

Place in a spot that is out of direct sunlight and let sit for 4 weeks. Check on this blend regularly. Be reminded of your intention and why you're making this medicine. Watch it. Smell it and taste it throughout its weeks of macerating.

After 4 weeks, strain, and if adding flower essences, you can add 2 to 5 drops now. Store in a labeled jar or dropper bottles.

TO USE

Take 1 full dropper (¼ teaspoon) one to three times a day, in water or tea, as needed.

HEART LOVE BATH + BODY OIL

Makes about 7 baths,
14–16 oz (415–480 ml) oil

There are many ways we can provide ourselves with love and self-care, such as taking a bath or giving ourselves a massage. Baths are a wonderful way to relax the nervous system and the heart and increase circulation. I like to use aromatic herbs such as rose, lemon balm and tulsi, especially when I'm looking to uplift the heart.

Creating herbal oils to use for self-massage is another wonderful way to ease stress, increase circulation, reduce heart rate and lower blood pressure. The scents of rose, vanilla and cinnamon are divine and nourishing to the nervous and circulatory system, not to mention the benefit our joints and skin also receive. So, if you have time, even if it's just once or twice a week, I highly suggest this as a wonderful act of self-love, self-care and stress reduction.

BATH

1 cup (25 g) dry or fresh lemon balm

1 cup (51 g) dry or fresh linden

¾ cup (9 g) dry or fresh rose petals

½ cup (10 g) dry or fresh tulsi

¼ cup (35 g) cinnamon chips

WHAT YOU'LL NEED FOR THE BATH

½-gal (2-L) jar

Cheesecloth

Rubber band or string

OIL

¾ cup (9 g) dried rose petals

¼ cup (5 g) dried tulsi (optional)

¼ cup (6 g) dried lemon balm (optional)

2 tbsp (16 g) cinnamon powder

1–2 vanilla beans

14–16 oz (390–455 g) coconut, olive or jojoba oil (or a blend of any of these)

WHAT YOU'LL NEED FOR THE OIL

Spice grinder

16-oz (480-ml) jar

Chopstick (optional)

Double boiler (optional)

Strainer

4 (2-oz [60-ml]) dropper bottles or a jar, for storage

TO MAKE THE HERBAL BATH

Gather your ingredients and measure out all the herbs into a mixing bowl. Using your hands, mix together until well blended. It will look and smell fabulous! Store in a ½-gallon (2-L) jar until ready to use.

Cut out a square piece of cheesecloth about 10" x 10" (25 x 25 cm) and place ¼ to ½ cup (10 to 20 g) of the bath blend in the center of the cloth. Gather all the ends and, using a rubber band or piece of string, wrap all the sides so the herbs are enclosed. Place in a running bath. You can also use this herb bundle as a body scrub.

TO MAKE THE OIL

Gather the herbs, except the vanilla beans, grind them one by one into a powder and place them into a 16-ounce (480-ml) jar. Next, slice the vanilla bean lengthwise, open it up and add to the jar.

Then fill the jar with your oil of choice. Cover and shake it around or mix the oil and herbs with a chopstick, making sure to get all the air bubbles out.

Label the jar and let the herbs sit for 4 weeks. Alternatively, for a faster option, you can place the herbs and oils in a double boiler and warm on the lowest heat for 2 to 4 hours. I like to make sure the oil never gets warmer than 100°F (38°C) to preserve the medicinal properties of the herbs.

Once the oil is done, strain it and store in a beautiful labeled bottle or dropper bottles. Massage the oil all over your body using upward motions, starting at the feet and moving in an upward direction toward the heart. Use liberally all over your body daily!

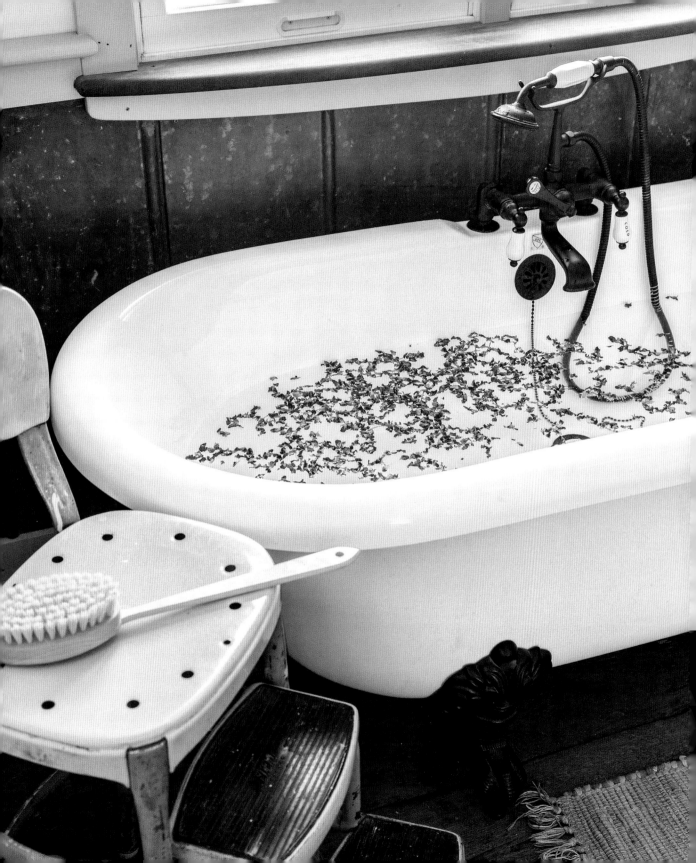

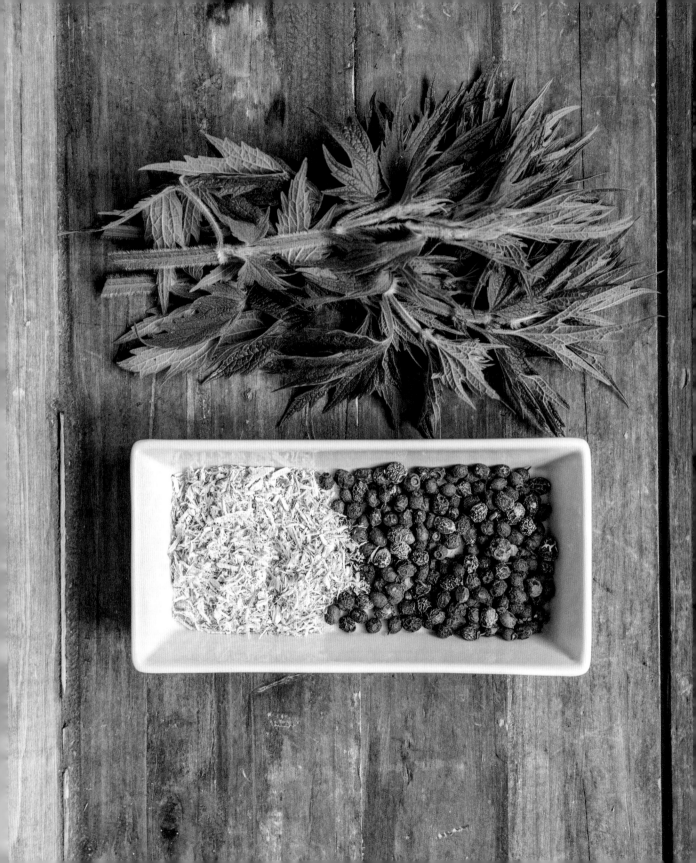

LIONHEARTED TINCTURE

Makes 6–8 oz (180–240 ml)

This formula is all about strengthening the heart, increasing circulation and helping either to prevent heart disease or to prevent it from developing further. This is a mighty blend made with herbs such as hawthorn berries, motherwort and astragalus root. Hawthorn is a cardio trophorestorative, which means it's nourishing and restoring to the heart and circulatory system, making it a fabulous herb to both support and nourish the functions of the heart and cardiovascular system. Motherwort is a favorite of mine to use for conditions with heart palpitations, and astragalus root is a cardiotonic and helps increase blood flow, making it great for supporting circulation.

TINCTURE

2 tbsp (21 g) dried hawthorn berries

1 tbsp (2 g) dried motherwort

1 tbsp (5 g) dried astragalus root

2 tsp (1 g) dried linden

2–4 tbsp (40–80 g) honey (optional)

About 1 cup (240 ml) vodka

OPTIONAL ADDITIONS

For Atherosclerosis

2 tsp (3 g) dried gingko biloba

1 tsp dried angelica

For High Cholesterol

2 tsp (8 g) dried burdock root

1 oz (30 ml) fresh milky oat tincture or 3 tbsp (4 g) fresh milky oat tops (see Note)

For Hypertension

1 tsp dried schisandra berries

2 tsp (3 g) dried passionflower

For Fluid Retention

1 tbsp (1 g) dried dandelion leaf

1 tsp yarrow

WHAT YOU'LL NEED

Spice grinder

8-oz (240-ml) jar

Strainer

4 (2-oz [60-ml]) dropper bottles or a jar, for storage

Gather all the herbs, including any of the optional ones you'd like to use. One by one, measure them out and run them through a spice grinder, then place into an 8-ounce (240-ml) jar. If you don't have a grinder, you can just measure out the herbs and place directly into the jar.

If using honey, you can add it now. Next, pour in the vodka until the jar is filled. Mix it all together and add more alcohol if needed, then place the cap on and shake. Open the jar back up and check to see if the alcohol level has dropped. If it has, add more to the jar and cover back up.

Label your jar and let sit for 4 weeks. Store in a place where you'll see it often. Shake it every week and taste a drop or two. After 4 weeks, strain and bottle in labeled 2-ounce (60-ml) dropper bottles or a jar.

TO USE

Take 1 full dropper (¼ teaspoon) once or twice a day, in water or tea.

Note: The High Cholesterol blend will be most effective using fresh milky oat tops. If you aren't able to source them fresh, you can purchase prepared fresh milky oat tincture from an herbal shop and use 1 ounce (30 ml) in this blend. Dried milky oat tops make a lovely infusion, but they don't come close to comparing to the medicinal activity of fresh milky oat tops when making a tincture. You can use an equal amount of dried, just be aware the tincture may not be as effective.

FIRE IT UP TEA

Yield varies

There are a lot of ways to turn up the heat, and this tea is one of them! If you're dealing with slow circulation, adding stimulating and circulating herbs such as ginger, cinnamon and cayenne to your diet is a great way to help boost blood flow. This tea makes a tasty addition to your tea pantry and is a good one to have around in the colder months.

INGREDIENTS

3 parts dried mint

1 part dried gingko biloba

½ part dried ginger pieces

½ part dried cinnamon chips

½ part dried yarrow flowers and leaf

Pinch of cayenne powder (optional)

WHAT YOU'LL NEED

Jar, for storage

Kettle

Strainer

First decide how much of the tea blend you'd like to make. I typically use cups for the parts so I have a large batch that will last me a few weeks or longer. If you'd like a smaller amount, use tablespoons, or use teaspoons for a single cup. Tablespoon measurements will give you about under ½ cup (23 g) of tea blend. If using cups, you'll get about 5½ cups (250 g) of tea blend.

Once you've chosen your measurements, gather the herbs and add them to a mixing bowl. Using your hands, mix the herbs together until well blended. Store in a jar.

To make a cup of tea, use 1½ teaspoons (1.5 g) per 1 cup (240 ml) of boiling water, then strain into a cup and enjoy!

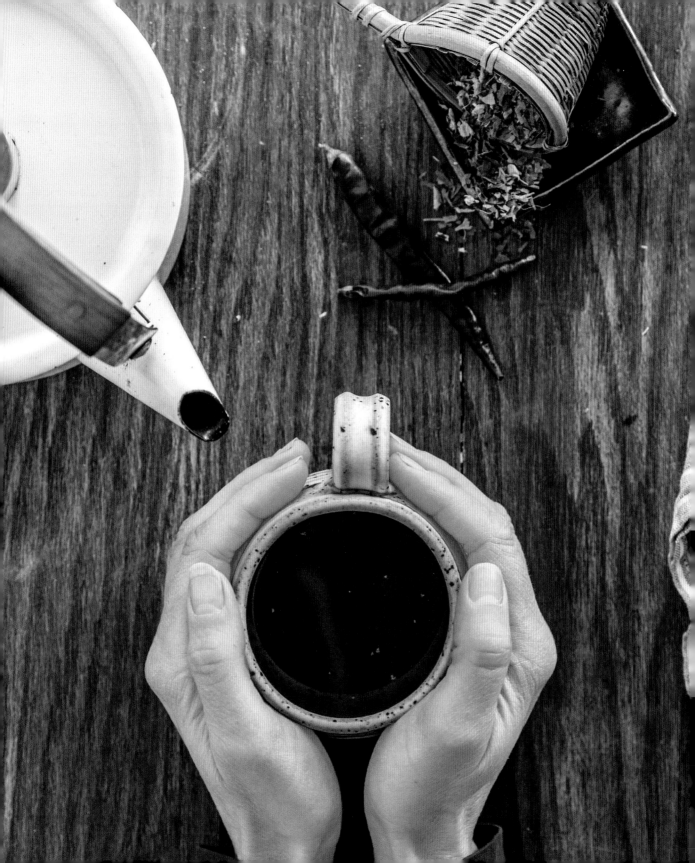

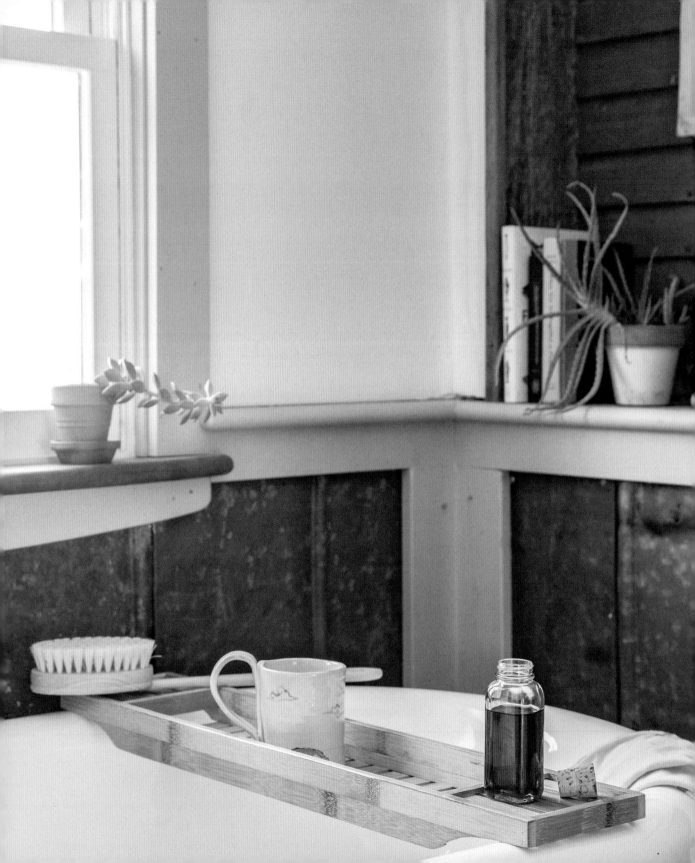

CIRCULATION BATH + BODY OIL

Makes 7 baths,
14–16 oz (415–480 ml) oil

My hands and feet struggle to stay warm in the wintertime. I spend a lot of time outdoors, and what better way to heat things back up when I get inside than an herbal bath? Fabulous herbs to use for supporting circulation are ginger, cinnamon and cayenne. Used together, they can especially bring warmth and circulation to the extremities of the hands and feet. You can also make this into a footbath or an oil. This oil can be used on areas that get cold and stiff. If you plan to use it on cold joints, then I would recommend using sesame oil; otherwise, olive oil or jojoba works well.

Always pay attention when working with a plant such as cayenne. You don't need much and be careful not to let it get into sensitive areas, as it can burn.

BATH

1 cup (93 g) dried ginger pieces

1 cup (144 g) dried cinnamon chips

⅓ cup (6 g) dried yarrow

2 tsp (7 g) cayenne powder

WHAT YOU'LL NEED FOR THE BATH

½-gal (2-L) jar

Cheesecloth

Rubber band or string

OIL

½ cup (45 g) dried ginger pieces

½ cup (67 g) dried cinnamon chips

¼ cup (5 g) dried yarrow

1 tbsp (10 g) cayenne powder

2 cups (480 ml) sesame, olive or jojoba oil (or a blend of any of these)

WHAT YOU'LL NEED FOR THE OIL

Spice grinder

16-oz (480-ml) jar

Chopstick (optional)

Double boiler (optional)

Strainer

4 (2-oz [60-ml]) dropper bottles or a jar, for storage

TO MAKE THE BATH

Gather your ingredients and, one by one, measure them into a mixing bowl. Using your hands, mix together until well blended. Store in a ½-gallon (2-L) jar until ready to use.

Cut a square piece of cheesecloth about 10" x 10" (25 x 25 cm) and place ¼ to ½ cup (27 to 54 g) of the bath blend in the center of the cloth. Gather all the ends and use a rubber band or piece of string to wrap all the side so the herbs are enclosed. Place in a running bath. You can also use this herb bundle as a body scrub.

TO MAKE THE OIL

Gather all the herbs. One by one, measure them out and run them through a spice grinder, grind them one by one into a powder and place them in the 16-oz (480-ml) jar. Since the cayenne is already in powder form, you can add it directly to the jar. If you don't have a grinder, you can just measure out the herbs and place directly into the jar.

Then fill the jar with your oil of choice. Cover and shake it around or mix the oil and herbs with a chopstick, making sure to get all the air bubbles out.

Label the jar and let the oil sit for 4 weeks. Alternatively, for a faster option, you can place the oil and herbs in a double boiler and warm on the lowest heat for 2 to 4 hours. I like to make sure the oil never gets warmer than 100°F (38°C) to preserve the medicinal properties of the herbs.

Once the oil is done, strain it and store in a labeled beautiful bottle or dropper bottles. Massage the oil all over your body using upward motions, starting at the feet and moving in an upward direction toward the heart. It's also great to use on cold hands, feet and joints.

"GIVE BEETS A CHANCE" SOUP WITH MUSHROOM + GARLIC STOCK

Makes 4 servings

I love growing, harvesting, eating and using beets. They're a wonderful food that grows and stores easily and for a long time. Whenever I eat beets, I always associate it with my blood and heart.

Beets are a powerful food, high in vitamin C, folate, vitamin B_6, magnesium, potassium, manganese, iron and nitrates. The high concentration of nitrates in beets has been shown to help lower blood pressure and lower the risk of heart attack and stroke. Making a simple soup with beets, mushrooms, astragalus and garlic is a wonderful and delicious way to support the heart, cardiovascular system and immune system.

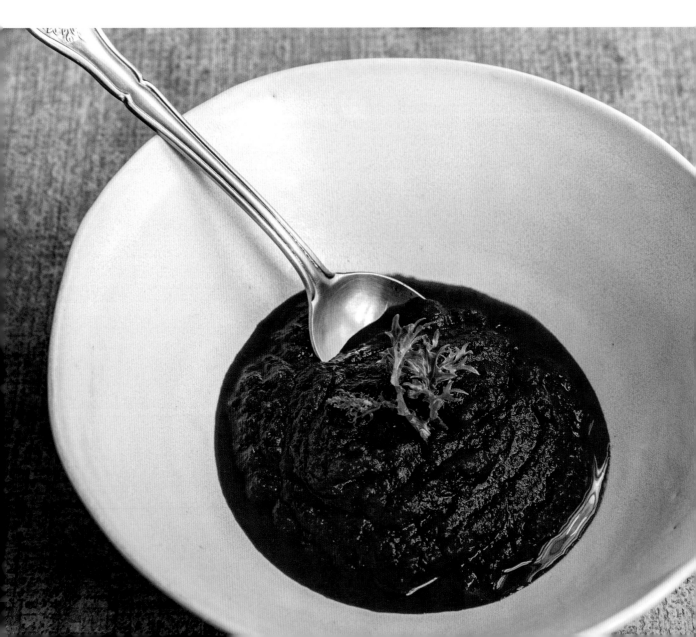

MUSHROOM + GARLIC STOCK

⅓–½ cup (10–13 g) dried reishi (pieces, slices or ground)

⅓–½ cup (10–13 g) dried maitake

2 tbsp (10 g) dried astragalus root

1 whole garlic bulb, cloves peeled and smashed

1 medium onion, roughly chopped

2 celery ribs with leaves, roughly chopped

1 cup (66 g) kale or kale ribs, roughly chopped

12 cups (3 L) water

WHAT YOU'LL NEED FOR THE STOCK

3-qt (3-L) pot

Strainer

1-qt (1-L) jar, for storage

SOUP

5 beets, diced

Olive oil as needed

1–2 tsp (6–12 g) sea salt

1 tsp black pepper, or to taste

1 tbsp (8 g) cumin powder

1 large onion, roughly chopped

1 whole garlic bulb, cloves peeled and smashed

1–2 tsp (3–6 g) smoked paprika or cayenne

2 cups (132 g) chopped kale

1½ cups (360 ml) Mushroom + Garlic Stock

½ cup (8 g) chopped fresh cilantro, for garnish

½ cup (73 g) roasted pumpkin seeds, for garnish

WHAT YOU'LL NEED FOR THE SOUP

2 roasting pans

Saucepan

Blender

TO MAKE THE STOCK

Place all the stock ingredients in a 3-quart (3-L) pot and bring to a boil over high heat. Once it's reached a boil, reduce the heat to a nice steady simmer and keep it there for at least 4 hours. You will need to add more water to the pot as the water reduces, but ultimately you are looking to yield about 6 cups (1.4 L) of stock after the 4 hours of simmering. When the stock is done cooking, strain 4 cups (960 ml) into a 1-quart (1-L) jar to store in the fridge or freezer, and set aside the remaining 2 cups (480 ml) for the soup.

TO MAKE THE SOUP

Preheat the oven to 425°F (220°C).

Spread out the diced beets on a roasting pan, drizzle with olive oil and sprinkle with a pinch of salt, a pinch of black pepper and cumin powder to taste. I *love* cumin. If cumin isn't your jam, then I would recommend trying fennel seeds. Use your hands to massage it all together until the beets are well coated, then set aside.

On a second roasting pan, place the onion and garlic. Drizzle with olive oil and sprinkle with a pinch of salt, a pinch of pepper and smoked paprika, and again massage it all together so it gets nice and coated.

Place the roasting pans in the oven and roast for about 15 minutes. After 15 minutes, check on them to see if the veggies might be done. The vegetables should be cooked through and almost caramelized.

While the vegetables are roasting, heat a pan with a little olive oil over medium-low heat and gently sauté the kale until it turns bright green and softens. Set aside.

Once the vegetables are done roasting, remove them from the oven. Place all the vegetables, including the sautéed kale right into a blender. Add the soup stock until it covers all the veggies, about 1 cup (240 ml). Blend for 1 to 3 minutes. From there, continue to slowly add more soup stock until the soup reaches a nice bisque-like consistency. If you want it thinner, keep adding stock.

Serve the soup in a lovely bowl garnished with the chopped cilantro and roasted pumpkin seeds. Yum!

HAWTHORN HEART SYRUP

Makes ½–¾ cup (120–180 ml)

Creating syrups with berries and herbs is a delicious way to turn medicine into food. Hawthorn is one of my favorite berries to work with in this way and combines well with other berries and herbs, such as goji berries and reishi.

Hawthorn is often used to help prevent atherosclerosis and relieve mild angina pain. Goji berries can be helpful for supporting circulation and preventing cold hands and feet. Reishi can help relieve angina pain, lower LDL cholesterol and blood pressure and support overall function of the cardiovascular system. Making this syrup is a fabulous way to offer love and support to the heart in the tastiest of ways. Hope you enjoy this one!

INGREDIENTS

¼ cup (25 g) hawthorn berries

¼ cup (33 g) blueberries

1 tbsp (9 g) goji berries

2 tsp (2 g) ground reishi

1–2 tbsp (8–16 g) grated fresh ginger

1–2 cinnamon sticks

4 cups (960 ml) boiling water

¼–½ cup (60–120 ml) maple syrup and/or honey

Zest of 1 lemon

⅛–¼ cup (30–60 ml) hawthorn tincture or brandy (optional)

WHAT YOU'LL NEED

Small pot with lid

Immersion blender or blender

Strainer

8-oz (240-ml) jar

Place the berries, reishi, ginger and cinnamon into a small pot, then pour the boiling water into the pot. Cover with a lid and let sit for 30 minutes or so.

After about 30 minutes, heat the pot over medium heat and let it come to a simmer. Once at a simmer, turn the heat down to low and let it cook for about 20 minutes.

After 20 minutes of cooking, turn off the heat and let sit again for 20 to 30 minutes. Do this process two or three more times. During this time if too much water is lost, then add more water back in.

Next, remove the cinnamon sticks from the pot and use an immersion blender in the pot (or transfer to a blender) to blend all the ingredients into a mash. If you used a blender, transfer the mash back to the pot. Place the cinnamon sticks back into the pot and continue cooking at a low simmer until the liquid has reduced to ½ cup (120 ml).

Once it's reduced to ½ cup (120 ml), strain off the herbs and cinnamon stick, pressing on the solids to extract as much liquid as possible, and place the liquid back into the pot. Add the maple syrup and lemon zest. You can start with ¼ cup (60 ml) of maple syrup, taste and then see if you want to add more for a sweeter syrup. If using, you can add the hawthorn tincture at this time to increase the shelf life.

Let the syrup cool completely. Place in a labeled bottle or jar and store in the fridge.

TO USE

Take one spoonful a day, either straight or added to oatmeal, pancakes, smoothies and pretty much any recipe that calls for maple syrup. You will notice that I use this recipe as the sweet component for a few other recipes in the book. So good.

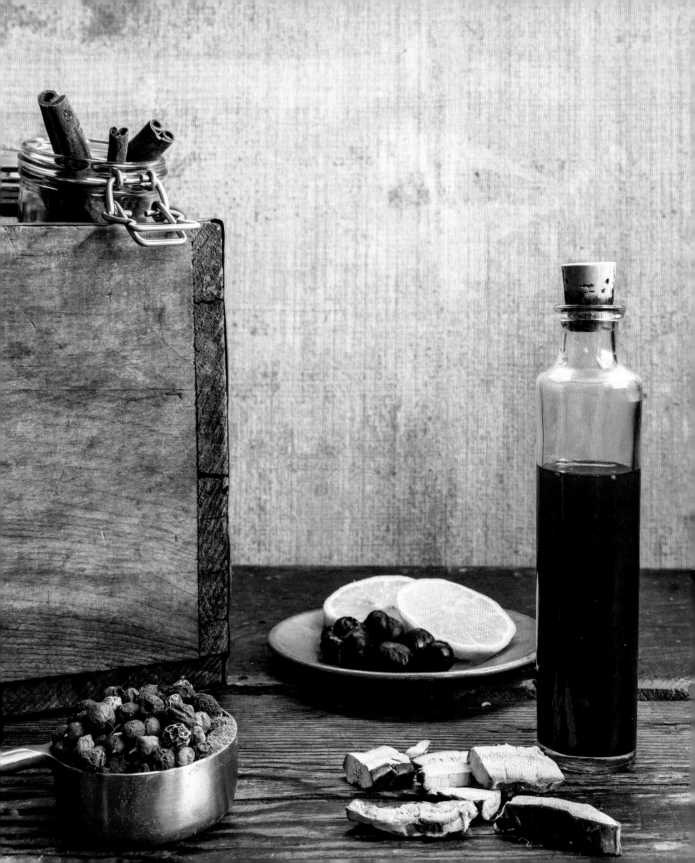

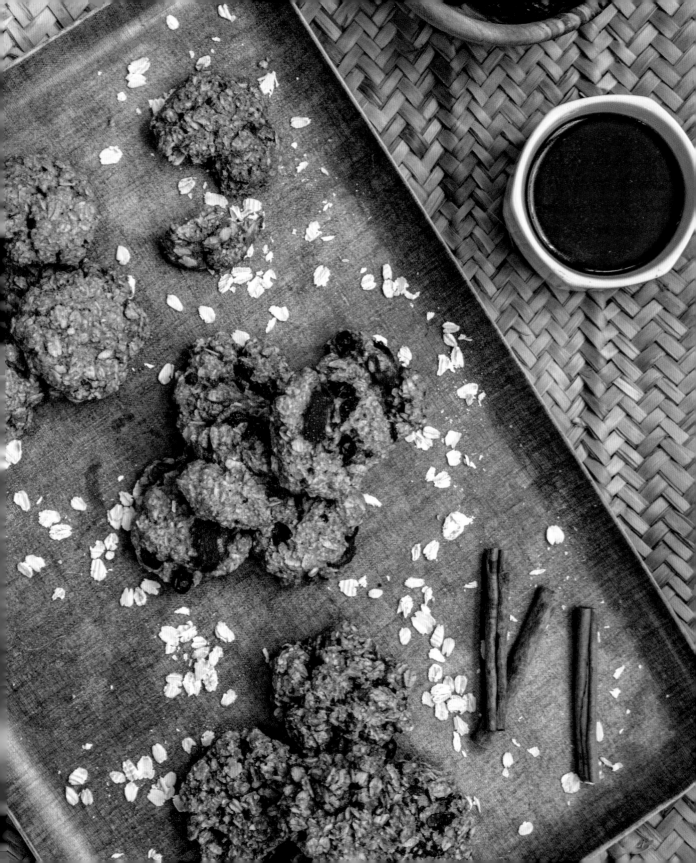

EAT YOUR HEART OUT COOKIES 3 WAYS

Makes 24 cookies

My mom, Pat, and I both enjoy a good healthy snack, but Gus, my partner, my dad, Ray, and my sister, Tara, all have a serious sweet tooth. So, I'm always looking for low-sugar, heart-healthy snacks and treats to make for my family. These cookies are made with heart-loving oats and cinnamon and they're sweetened with the Hawthorn Heart Syrup on page 126.

Oats are beneficial in lowering LDL cholesterol and blood pressure, and they're high in antioxidants. Cinnamon is delicious and can help lower blood pressure and increase circulation. Ashwagandha is a great adaptogen that can be helpful for fatigue. I've included three different variation ideas for add-ins, but play around and have fun coming up with your own versions.

COOKIES

⅓ cup (80 g) coconut oil

1 tsp ashwagandha powder

1 cup (128 g) oat flour

1½ cups (168 g) rolled oats

1 tsp baking powder

⅓ tsp sea salt

1½ tsp (5 g) cinnamon powder

1 egg

1½ tsp (7 ml) vanilla extract

¼–⅓ cup (60–80 ml) Hawthorn Heart Syrup (page 126) or maple syrup

BREAKFAST ADD-INS

¼ cup (35 g) fresh/frozen blueberries

¼ cup (35 g) fresh/frozen strawberries

LUNCH ADD-INS

Handful chopped chocolate

Handful chopped pecans

DINNER ADD-INS

1–2 tbsp (8–16 g) grated fresh ginger

WHAT YOU'LL NEED

Saucepan

2 baking sheets

Parchment paper

Preheat the oven to 350°F (180°C).

Add the coconut oil to a small saucepan and warm it over low heat. While it's heating, measure out the ashwagandha, add to the oil and let it slowly warm. Once it's all melted and mixed together, set it aside.

Next, combine the oat flour, oats, baking powder, salt and cinnamon in a small bowl. In a separate large mixing bowl, whisk the egg. Add the vanilla, hawthorn syrup and ashwagandha–coconut oil mixture and whisk together until combined. Once the wet ingredients are nicely mixed, slowly add in the dry ingredients.

Now here's where it gets fun. You can divide the batter into thirds in three different bowls. Add the extra ingredients to each bowl and mix well.

If the batter is soft, you can chill it in the fridge for 10 to 15 minutes; otherwise, you can get to baking!

Line two baking sheets with parchment paper. Using a spoon or tablespoon, scoop the batter into rounded tablespoon-size balls and place onto the sheets. Bake for 12 to 15 minutes. Watch the cookies toward the end of the baking time. They should be golden on the edges and on top, and soft in the center. You can adjust the sizes to what you like, just adjust the baking time accordingly. Enjoy!

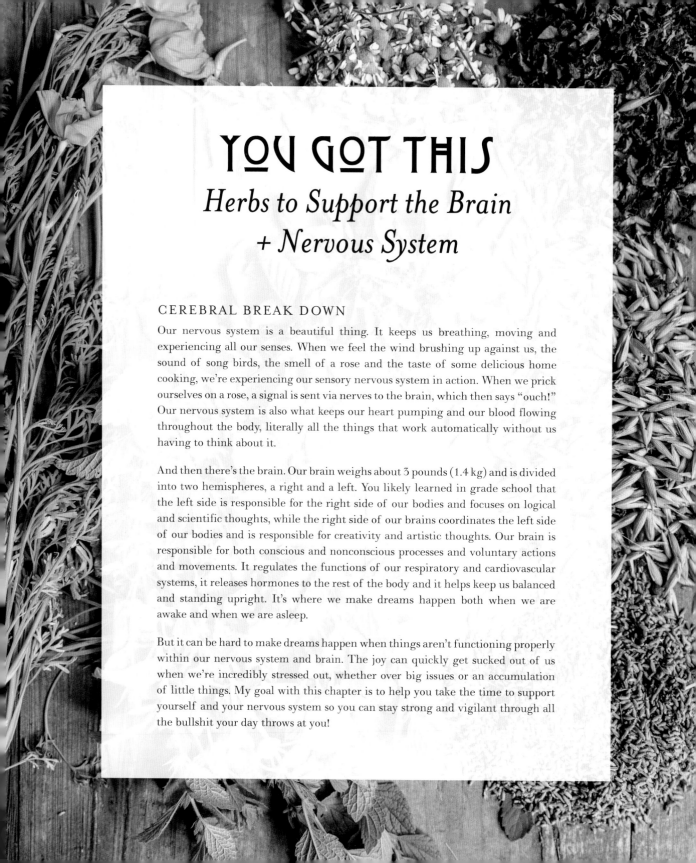

YOU GOT THIS
Herbs to Support the Brain + Nervous System

CEREBRAL BREAK DOWN

Our nervous system is a beautiful thing. It keeps us breathing, moving and experiencing all our senses. When we feel the wind brushing up against us, the sound of song birds, the smell of a rose and the taste of some delicious home cooking, we're experiencing our sensory nervous system in action. When we prick ourselves on a rose, a signal is sent via nerves to the brain, which then says "ouch!" Our nervous system is also what keeps our heart pumping and our blood flowing throughout the body, literally all the things that work automatically without us having to think about it.

And then there's the brain. Our brain weighs about 3 pounds (1.4 kg) and is divided into two hemispheres, a right and a left. You likely learned in grade school that the left side is responsible for the right side of our bodies and focuses on logical and scientific thoughts, while the right side of our brains coordinates the left side of our bodies and is responsible for creativity and artistic thoughts. Our brain is responsible for both conscious and nonconscious processes and voluntary actions and movements. It regulates the functions of our respiratory and cardiovascular systems, it releases hormones to the rest of the body and it helps keep us balanced and standing upright. It's where we make dreams happen both when we are awake and when we are asleep.

But it can be hard to make dreams happen when things aren't functioning properly within our nervous system and brain. The joy can quickly get sucked out of us when we're incredibly stressed out, whether over big issues or an accumulation of little things. My goal with this chapter is to help you take the time to support yourself and your nervous system so you can stay strong and vigilant through all the bullshit your day throws at you!

As I've said in many other chapters, but is so important it's worth driving home, one thing that can have an impact on improving the health of our nervous system is removing processed foods and white sugars from our diet. The brain-to-gut connection is powerful, and eating foods that are prebiotic and probiotic can be beneficial to our mood. Movement has shown to reduce stress levels and increase dopamine—the happy hormone. Go to an animal shelter and walk a dog or just curl up with a bunch of cats. Spending time with animals is a wonderful way to lower stress, and the research is there to back it up. Decrease caffeine. If you're experiencing anxiety or panic attacks, caffeine can truly be like throwing fuel on a fire. Healthy fats, omega-3s, B vitamins, vitamin D and, of course, herbs can all be beneficial things to add to your diet.

We can do a lot with herbs to help reduce our daily stress. Wonderful herbs that can help support our nervous system and alleviate mild depression and anxiety include but are not exclusive to lemon balm, passionflower, fresh milky oat tops, tulsi, ashwagandha and reishi.

SLEEP

Sleep is such an important part of our day. This is a place and time when our bodies are able to heal and restore themselves. If we don't get enough sleep, there are a whole host of issues that can arise, such as depression, anxiety, high blood pressure, stroke, heart attack, digestive issues, obesity and diabetes.

The average adult should be getting seven to nine hours of sleep each night, and it's even better if we go to bed and wake up at about the same time every day. Unfortunately, sleep can be a great challenge for people for numerous reasons, such as stress, anxiety, working the late shift or swing shifts and illness. Symptoms of stress on the nervous system or endocrine system can result in sleep disturbances or insomnia. It's important to look closely at what the root cause of this might be while also supporting the body with herbs that can help support sleep. Some of my favorite go-to herbs to help support sleep issues are California poppy, passionflower, skullcap, lavender, chamomile and milky oat tops.

Something to consider is to remove coffee from your diet if you're experiencing sleep issues, panic attacks or anxiety. Coffee is wonderfully delicious, but it can be overstimulating if you have anxiety or sleep issues, so we offer a great coffee alternative: Roasted Roots Herbal Coffee on page 24. Also, again, watch the foods you eat and limit alcohol consumption and any stimulating drugs.

GETTING THROUGH THE HAZE

As we get older, being "in a haze" might not mean the same thing it did when we were in our twenties. There are a lot of health issues that can cloud our thoughts and create a fog, making it challenging to think clearly. Besides stress, other things can cause brain fog are hormones, illness, food allergies or sensitivities and injuries.

It's important to pay close attention to what you're eating. Always. Once you start paying attention, you may notice a connection between symptoms showing up and something you ate a few hours earlier. There are a lot of weird things in processed foods that can affect our brain, nervous system and pretty much everything else in our bodies.

As I said, there are a number of factors that can cause brain fog, so start doing a little detective work. Maybe you need some herbs that support the nervous system, brain and hormone balance. In this chapter, I include a wonderful all-around brain tonic (Clarity Elixir, page 145). However, you should definitely work on trying to figure out the source of this issue if you don't already know and then consider seeing a clinical herbalist, ND or other health practitioner to understand what's going on and how to create the best treatment plan for you.

Some great herbs you can add to your daily routine to address brain fog include rosemary, tulsi, bacopa, gotu kola, hawthorn, gingko biloba and lion's mane mushroom.

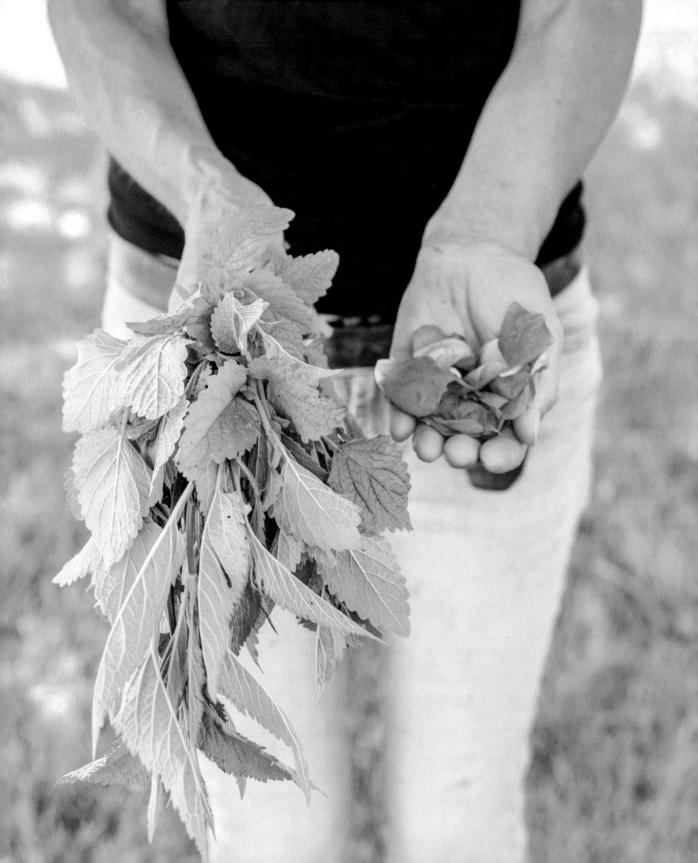

HANG IN THERE ELIXIR

Makes 6–8 oz (180–240 ml)

This is an antianxiety blend made with herbs such as rose, tulsi and lemon balm, which are anxiolytics, antidepressants, nervines and hormone balancers. This blend of herbs works on supporting our nervous system on a long-term basis while also supporting more acute needs.

Fresh milky oat tincture, or the actual fresh milky oat tops, is an important part of this formula. Fresh milky oat tops are a very specific ingredient and one that may be challenging for you to have on hand. Fresh milky oat tops are oats, such as oatmeal, that are harvested during a milky phase, which occurs right before the seed heads develop fully into seeds. Considered a trophorestorative for the nervous system, it's best tinctured fresh. So, how do you get your own fresh milky oat tincture? Oats are easy to grow and can even be grown in pots. You can harvest the tops when ready, make into a fresh tincture and have it on hand. You can also purchase some prepared tincture from a local herbalist to use in this elixir. Dried milky oat tops make a lovely infusion, but they don't come close to comparing to the medicinal activity of fresh milky oat tops when making a tincture. You could use an equal amount of dried, but the tincture will not be nearly as effective.

INGREDIENTS

4 tbsp (60 ml) fresh milky oat tincture or 6 tbsp (8 g) fresh milky oat tops (see headnote)

2 tbsp (8 g) dried passionflower

2 tbsp (3 g) dried lemon balm

1 tbsp (1 g) dried rose petals

1 tbsp (2 g) dried tulsi

1 tsp dried blue vervain

1–2 tbsp (20–40 g) honey (optional)

About 1 cup (240 ml) vodka

WHAT YOU'LL NEED

Spice grinder

8-oz (240-ml) jar

Strainer

4 (2-oz [60-ml]) dropper bottles or a jar, for storage

When making medicine, holding intent and vision is an important part of the process, making it sacred. As you're gathering your herbs, meditate on why you're making this elixir. This is a powerful aspect to making medicine, being clear with intent and putting our energy into it. Hold your reasons for making this medicine close to you while going through the following steps.

Gather all the herbs (including fresh milky oat tops, if using) and one by one measure them out and run them through a spice grinder, then place into an 8-ounce (240-ml) jar. If you don't have a grinder you can just measure out the herbs and place directly into the jar.

If using honey, you can add it now. Next, pour in the vodka until the jar is filled. Mix it all together and add more alcohol if needed, then place the cap on and shake. Open the jar back up and check to see if the alcohol level has dropped. If it has, add more to the jar and cover back up.

Label your jar and let sit for 4 weeks. Store in a place where you'll see it often. Shake it every week and taste a drop or two. After 4 weeks, strain and add the fresh milky oat tincture (if using) to the blend. Bottle in labeled 2-ounce (60-ml) dropper bottles or a jar.

TO USE

Take 1 full dropper (¼ teaspoon) one to three times a day in water or tea. This blend can also be used acutely. Take a dropperful or two if you are starting to feel the triggers of some anxiety, panic or depression come on and do this up to three times a day.

LOVE YOURSELF BODY OIL

Makes 16 oz (480 ml)

Massage is a wonderful way to reduce stress and anxiety, increase circulation, promote sound sleep and lower blood pressure. While dealing with Lyme disease, I had symptoms of heart palpitations and anxiety. To help decrease my symptoms, I gave myself a daily massage to help support and relax my nervous system, and it worked. Daily massage with an herbal oil is a wonderful act of self-love, self-care and stress reduction. This fabulous blend of roses, vanilla and cinnamon will relax and soothe your senses and nervous system. Enjoy!

INGREDIENTS

⅓ cup (6 g) dried rose petals

2 tbsp (21 g) cinnamon chips

2 tbsp (4 g) dried tulsi

2 tbsp (3 g) dried lemon balm

1 vanilla bean

2 cups (480 ml) olive, jojoba or coconut oil (or a blend)

WHAT YOU'LL NEED

16-oz (480-ml) jar

Strainer

8 (2-oz [60-ml]) dropper bottles or a jar, for storage

Gather all the herbs and measure them into a 16-ounce (480-ml) jar. Slice the vanilla bean lengthwise, open it up and add to the jar and then cover with the oil. Label the jar and let sit for 2 to 4 weeks. After 2 to 4 weeks, strain it and store in labeled 2-ounce (60-ml) dropper bottles or a jar.

TO USE
Massage all over the body.

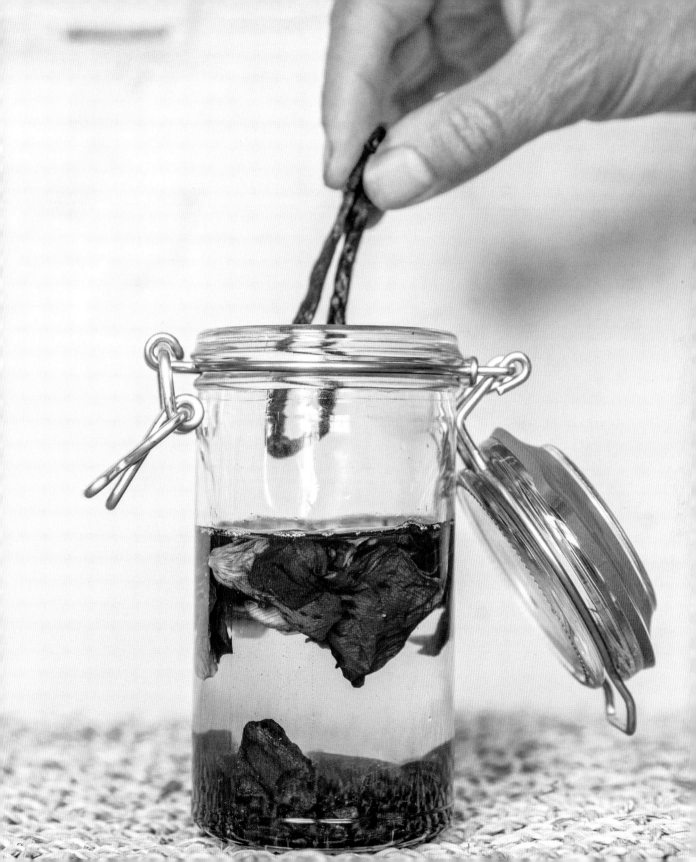

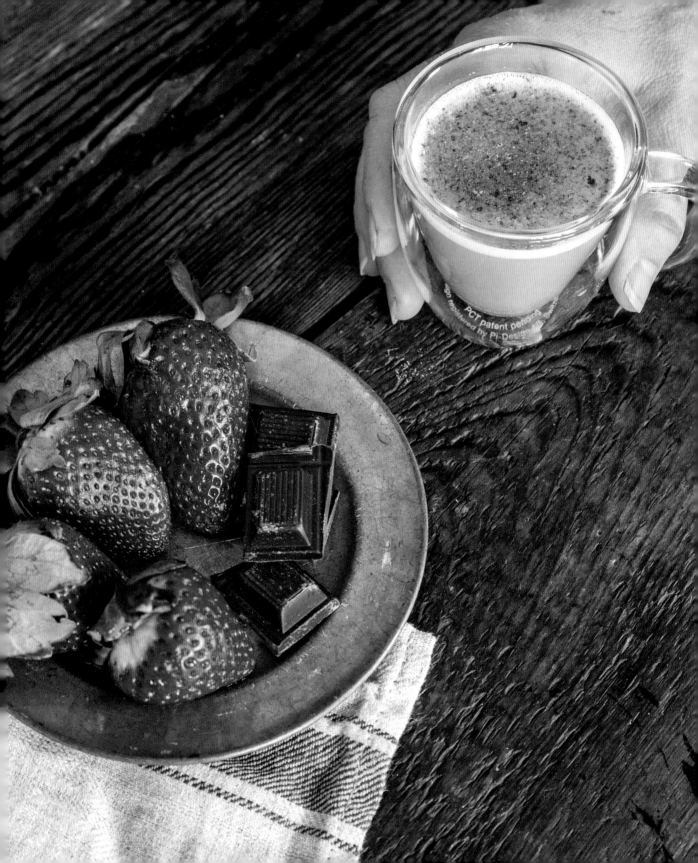

TULSI + ROSE TEA LATTE

Makes 1 serving

I love all of Herbal Revolution's products, but I especially love making the Tulsi + Rose Tea. The way it smells, the way it looks, the way it tastes—I love it all. This tea will make you feel so good just being around it! Vibrant, delicious rose and tulsi support the nervous system and are light and refreshing. Blending them with coconut cream gives this tea that little bit of cooling richness while still keeping it light. The beautiful appearance of this drink pairs well with the refreshing flavors and intent to show ourselves some love.

We live incredibly busy lives, which can make it challenging to stop and take a moment for ourselves. So, when we do, we should make it a good moment, a moment that feels indulgent and sacred. This latte is just the thing.

INGREDIENTS

2 tbsp (4 g) dried tulsi

1½ tbsp (2 g) dried lemon balm or lemon verbena

1 tbsp (2 g) dried milky oat tops or oat straw

2 tsp (1 g) dried rose petals, divided

2–3 dried cardamom pods

1 (13.5-oz [400-ml]) can coconut milk

Honey, to taste (optional)

WHAT YOU'LL NEED

16-oz (480-ml) jar

Kettle

Spice grinder

Whisk

Strainer

Blender or immersion blender

TO MAKE THE HERB BLEND

In a bowl, combine the tulsi, lemon balm, milky oat tops and 1 teaspoon (0.5 g) of the rose petals. Blend with your hands or a spoon. Once it's thoroughly mixed, take a moment to look at how beautiful the blend is and appreciate how lovely it smells.

TO MAKE THE LATTE

Place 2 teaspoons (2 g) of the herb blend in a jar, pour 1 cup (240 ml) of boiling water over the herbs and cover. Let steep for 5 to 10 minutes.

While the tea is steeping, grind the remaining 1 teaspoon (0.5 g) of rose petals in a spice grinder into a lovely powder. Do the same with the cardamom pods.

Open the can of coconut milk, pour it into a bowl and whisk until the thick cream and thinner liquid are evenly combined.

Once the tea is done steeping, strain and measure out ¾ cup (180 ml) of tea and place in a blender. Add ¼ cup (60 ml) of the coconut milk to the blender. If using honey, add it too and blend on medium-high speed for 30 seconds. Pour into a mug and sprinkle the top with the powdered rose and cardamom. Enjoy!

RELAX HONEY + INFUSION

Makes 8 oz (225 g) honey,
infusion yield varies

I'm always amazed at how much a cup of tea or a tea infusion can bring my nervous system back into balance. I believe that slowing down to make the tea blend and the tea is all part of the medicine. There is great beauty in combining herbs, especially relaxing and soothing herbs such as linden flower, rose and milky oat tops. Linden is a wonderful herb for treating anxiety and irritability, rose petals are uplifting to the spirit and can help with stagnant depression and anxiety, and milky oat tops are wonderful for the nervous system, helping with anxiety and for when we're feeling wired and tired. This blend can be enjoyed as a quick tea, but I think it's best to let it steep longer into an infusion. It's also delicious iced! This recipe is in two parts. There is an infused honey component, which is delicious, that can be made ahead of time and added to the infusion. Enjoy this one.

HONEY

3 tbsp (3 g) dried rose petals

2 tbsp (3 g) dried lemon balm

2 tbsp (4 g) dried milky oat tops

1 tbsp (3 g) dried tulsi

1 tbsp (4 g) dried linden flower

1 tsp dried ashwagandha powder

¾ cup (240 g) honey

WHAT YOU'LL NEED FOR THE HONEY

Spice grinder

8-oz (240-ml) jar

Strainer

Jar or bottles, for storage

INFUSION

3 parts dried milky oat tops

2 parts dried lemon balm

1 part dried passionflower

½ part dried tulsi

½ part dried rose petals

½ part dried mint (optional)

WHAT YOU'LL NEED FOR THE INFUSION

Storage jar

Kettle

French press or 1-qt (1-L) jar

Strainer

TO MAKE THE HONEY
Gather your herbs and one by one, measure them out and run them through a spice grinder, then place into an 8-ounce (240-ml) jar. If you don't have a grinder, you can just measure out the herbs and place directly into the jar. Add the honey. Stir it all together until well combined. Label the jar and let sit out on a warm or sunny countertop for 2 to 4 weeks. After 2 to 4 weeks, you can use as is or strain out the herbs, then bottle in a labeled jar.

TO USE THE HONEY
You can add the honey to hot water or any tea (especially the infusion below), or do what I do—just eat it straight.

TO MAKE THE INFUSION
First decide how much of the herb blend you'd like to make. I use cups for the parts, which makes about 7 cups (180 g) of the blend, so I have a large batch that will last me a couple of weeks. If you're looking to make just a couple of cups of infusion or tea, then I suggest using tablespoon measurements, which will give you about ½ cup (14 g) of blend.

Once you've figured out how much you want to make, start measuring the herbs into a mixing bowl. Use your hands to mix the herbs until it all comes together into a lovely, cohesive blend. Store in a jar until ready to use.

In a kettle, bring 4 cups (960 ml) of water to a boil. Place ¼ to ½ cup (7 to 14 g) of the blend in the French press, then add a spoonful of the infused honey. You can use more or less of the honey, depending on your taste. Fill the French press with boiling water and let steep for at least 2 hours and up to 12 hours before straining and drinking. If steeping overnight, you can leave it at room temperature. Or to make an iced tea you can put it in the fridge and enjoy it over ice the next day.

If you'd like to make a single cup of tea instead of the infusion, use 1 to 2 teaspoons (0.5 to 1 g) of herb blend per 1 cup (240 ml) of boiling water and steep for 5 to 15 minutes.

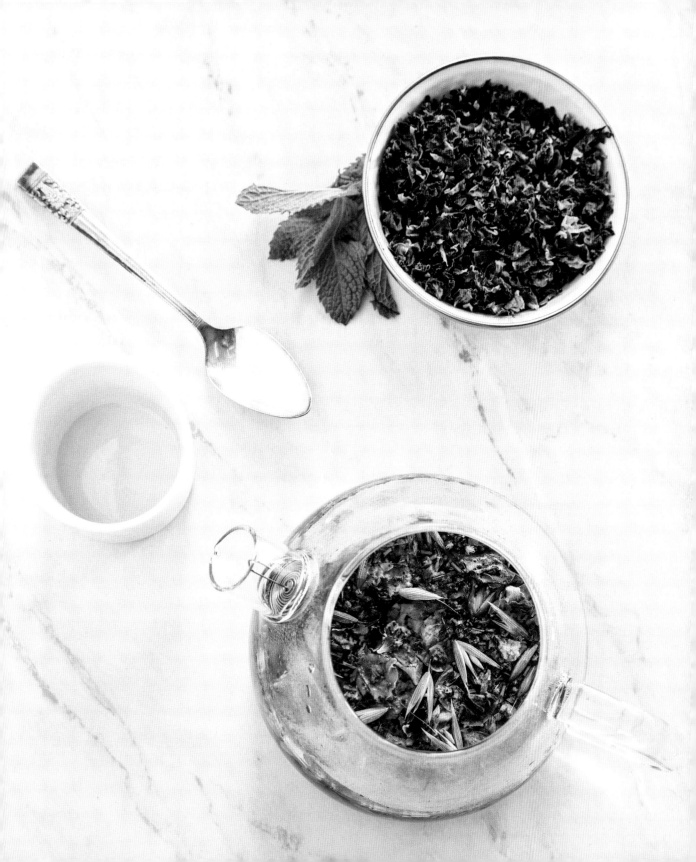

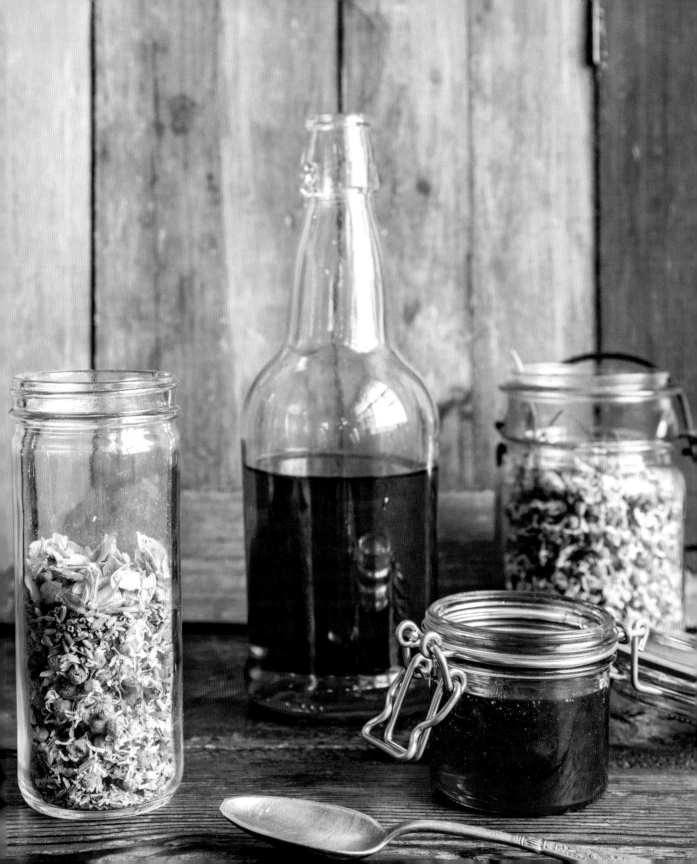

SLEEP ELIXIR

Makes 6–8 oz (180–240 ml)

We all need to sleep, but unfortunately, it's not always that easy. Issues such as stress, hormones, digestive problems, anxiety or working the night shift can all have an effect on our sleep. It's important to try and figure out the root cause of your sleeplessness, but while you're figuring it out, there are some herbs that can help support you.

This tincture is made with California poppy, passionflower and hops—these herbs are great sedatives and nervines. I love growing California poppy and looking out on the fields of golden orange blossoms. It can be helpful for insomnia that is accompanied by anxiety. Passionflower, another stunning flower, is wonderful for people who struggle to sleep because they can't shut their brains off. I also love hops, and especially love harvesting the beautiful strobiles. Hops can be beneficial for sleep issues induced by stress, PMS or menopause.

INGREDIENTS

2 tbsp (7 g) dried passionflower

1 tbsp (2 g) dried chamomile

1 tbsp (4 g) dried California poppy

1 tbsp (9 g) dried ashwagandha

1 tsp dried hops

1 tsp dried lavender (optional)

2–4 tbsp (40–80 g) honey (optional)

About 1 cup (240 ml) vodka

WHAT YOU'LL NEED

Spice grinder

8-oz (240 ml) jar

Strainer

4 (2-oz [60-ml]) dropper bottles or a jar, for storage

When making medicine, holding intent and vision is an important part of the process, especially with this blend for healing the emotional and the physical. As you're gathering your herbs, meditate on why you're making this elixir, whether it's for yourself, a family member or a friend in need. Holding your reasons for making this medicine close to you while going through the following steps is a powerful part of the medicine making.

Gather your herbs and one by one measure them out and run them through a spice grinder, then place them in an 8-ounce (240-ml) jar. If you don't have a grinder, you can just measure out the herbs and place directly into the jar.

If using honey, you can add it now. Next, pour in the vodka until the jar is filled. Mix everything together and add more vodka if needed to top off the jar. Then place the cap on and shake. Open the jar back up and check to see if the alcohol level has dropped. If it has, add more to the jar and cover back up.

Label the jar and let sit for 4 weeks. Store it in a place where you'll see it often. Shake it every week and taste a drop or two. After 4 weeks, strain and bottle into 2-ounce (60-ml) dropper bottles or a jar.

TO USE

Take 1 full dropper (¼ teaspoon) in water or tea after dinner and then again before bed. Preferably, if you feel your body naturally starting to become tired, stop using your computer, your phone or the TV. Take the tincture and head off to bed. You can also leave it on the nightstand and take a dropperful if you wake up in the night and have trouble getting back to sleep.

SWEET DREAMS TEA

Yield varies

This enchanting blend is made with herbs such as mugwort, lavender and catnip, which can help induce sweet dreams and keep nightmares at bay. Mugwort is a magical plant that is a nervine and often used for dreamwork. It helps guide us to the dream world while keeping out bad dreams and nightmares. Lavender is a lovely nervine that is helpful for inducing sleep, and catnip is a gentle sedative. All the herbs in this blend help calm and support our nervous system, while also working on an energetic and magical level. Plus, the act of preparing a warm cup of tea before bed can be very calming! This tea can be used in conjunction with the Sleep Elixir (page 141).

INGREDIENTS

3 parts dried catnip

2 parts dried skullcap

1 part dried chamomile

½ part dried lavender

½ part dried mugwort

WHAT YOU'LL NEED

Jar, for storage

Strainer

Kettle

First decide how much of the tea blend you'd like to make. I typically use cups for the parts so I have a large batch that will last me a few weeks or longer. If using cups, you'll get about 7 cups (150 g) of tea blend. If you'd like a smaller amount, use tablespoons, or use teaspoons for a single cup. Tablespoon measurements will give you about ½ cup (10 g) of tea blend.

Once you've chosen your measurements, measure the herbs layer by layer into a mixing bowl.

Use your hands to mix the herbs until it all comes together into a lovely, cohesive blend. Store in a jar until ready to use.

Make a cup of tea in the evening before bed. Use 1 to 1½ teaspoons (0.5 to 1 g) of herb blend per 1 cup (240 ml) of boiling water. Let steep for 5 to 10 minutes, then strain into your favorite mug and enjoy. Wishing you the sweetest dreams.

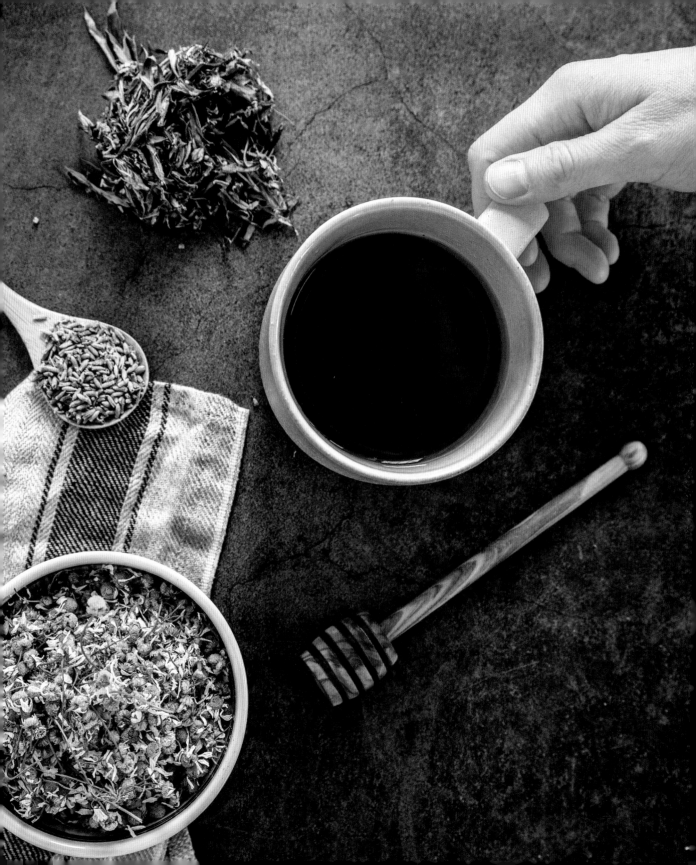

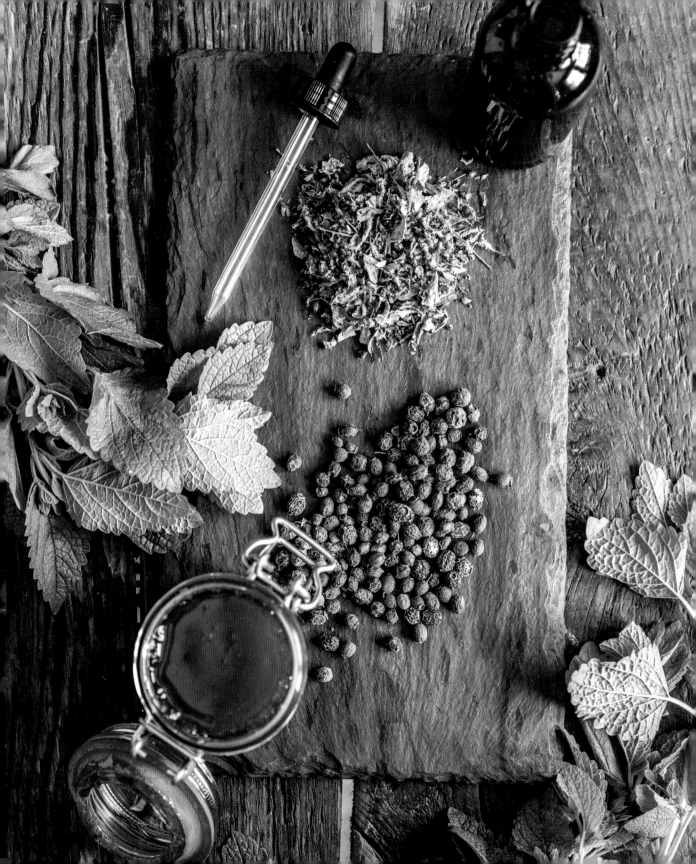

CLARITY ELIXIR

Makes 6–8 oz (180–240 ml)

There are often moments when we need more clarity, especially when going through times of stress, anxiety, depression, digestive issues, hormone changes and so much more. All of these things affect our nervous system and ultimately our minds. The fog sets in and some days it can be really thick. This formula is made with tulsi, rosemary and lemon balm to help us through those times of heavy haze. Tulsi is an herb I love using as a brain tonic. It can help clear and sharpen the mind, while also keeping both the body and the mind calm and relaxed. Rosemary is a lovely brain stimulant, bringing warmth and circulation to the brain, making it a wonderful fog lifter. Lemon balm is one of my go-to herbs for helping to uplift the spirit and combat any anxiety that might be part of the issue.

INGREDIENTS

1 tbsp (2 g) dried lemon balm

1 tbsp (3 g) dried tulsi

½ tsp dried rosemary

2 tsp (8 g) dried hawthorn

1 tsp dried ashwagandha

2–4 tbsp (40–80 g) honey (optional)

About 1 cup (240 ml) vodka

WHAT YOU'LL NEED

Spice grinder

8-oz (240-ml) jar

Strainer

4 (2-oz [60-ml]) dropper bottles or a jar, for storage

Gather your herbs and one by one, measure them out and run them through a spice grinder, then place into an 8-ounce (240-ml) jar. If you don't have a grinder, you can just measure out the herbs and place directly into the jar.

If using honey, you can add it now. Next, pour in the vodka until the jar is filled. Stir the herbs around in the jar and add more vodka if needed to top off the jar. Then place the cap on and shake. Open the jar back up and check to see if the alcohol level has dropped. If it has, add more to the jar and cover back up.

Label the jar and let sit for 4 weeks. Store in a place where you'll see it often. Shake it every week and taste a drop or two. After 4 weeks, you can strain and bottle into labeled 2-ounce (60-ml) dropper bottles or a jar.

TO USE

Take 1 full dropper (¼ teaspoon) one to three times a day, in water or tea, as needed.

BEAUTIFUL + BRILLIANT BRAIN BITES

Makes 24 balls

Back in the day, I used to make ganja goo balls and sling them on the lot at Grateful Dead shows. I've since adapted my twenty-five-year-old recipe to focus on herbs and nuts that are tonics for the brain. Nuts are high in vitamin E, antioxidants and healthy fats—all things that our brains love. The herbs in this blend, especially bacopa, eleuthero and rhodiola, are adaptogens, nervines and brain tonics. Healthy circulation in our brains is a must if we want to be brilliant, so using nootropics such as bacopa regularly can help promote cerebral circulation, boost memory, uplift our mood and slow down cognitive decline. Eleuthero is an adaptogen that is often used for cognitive function, alertness and stress. Rhodiola is also an adaptogen that can help improve memory, boost mood and lessen fatigue.

I hope you enjoy these tasty bites as much as I do. Please feel free to mix and match using different nuts and seed butters.

INGREDIENTS

1 cup (118 g) rolled oats (quick oats can work too)

2 tsp (6 g) dried eleuthero powder

2 tsp (6 g) dried rhodiola powder

2 tsp (6 g) dried bacopa powder

1 tsp dried ashwagandha powder

2 tbsp (20 g) goji berries

1 tbsp (10 g) cacao nibs

1 cup (240 g) nut butter (I like to use either chunky peanut butter or almond butter)

⅛–½ cup (40–160 g) honey, to taste

¼ cup (35 g) sesame seeds

¼ cup (38 g) ground pecan meal

¼ cup (17 g) unsweetened shredded coconut

WHAT YOU'LL NEED

Parchment paper

Storage container

Place the oats, eleuthero, rhodiola, bacopa, ashwagandha, goji berries and cacao nibs in a bowl. Using a spoon or fork, mix them all together. Add the nut butter and honey and mix until it all comes together in a nice smooth dough. If it seems too gooey, you can add more oats; if it's too dry you can add more nut butter and/or honey if you want it sweeter.

Place the sesame seeds, ground pecan meal and shredded coconut into separate shallow bowls to use for rolling the balls.

Using a tablespoon measure or spoon, scoop the mixture and form it into a ball in your hands. Roll and cover the ball in your choice of sesame seeds, pecan meal or shredded coconut. Set on a piece of parchment paper to harden and repeat until all of the mixture is gone. Store in an airtight container in the fridge for up to 2 weeks.

These are so good! And easy to eat all at once. I recommend 1 to 4 balls a day for brain support.

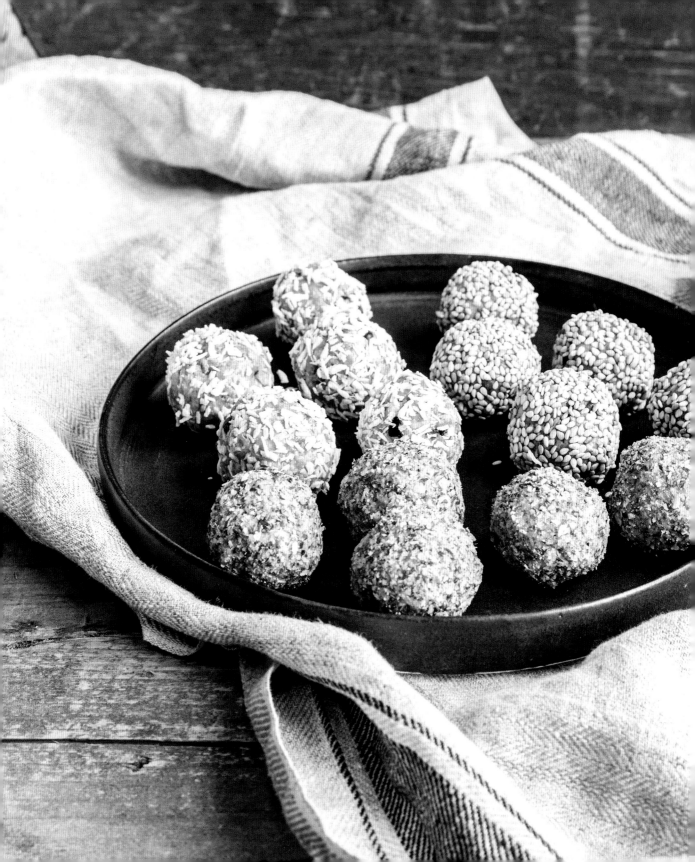

STRENGTH + BEAUTY FROM THE INSIDE OUT
Supporting Skin, Muscles + Bones

WE'RE MORE THAN JUST SKIN AND BONES

I was around nineteen years old, working at the Belfast Co-op, when my manager, Jill, gave me a book on how to make herbal body products. At this point, I already had a small handful of herbal books by Rosemary Gladstar and Deb Soule, and I was so grateful to add another book to my growing collection.

As soon as Jill gave me that book on body care, I set off to make my first body product, a Lilac Body Cream for my mémère, whose favorite flower was lilac. That was almost twenty-five years ago, and I remember it so clearly: the gorgeous spring day, the farmhouse I lived in, the cream, which came out pretty good for my first try, and my mémère loving it. Since those early days, I've gone on to study the body more in depth and create many different types of topical products for supporting the skin and easing muscle and nerve aches and pains.

Our skin is the largest organ of the body: It can weigh 6 to 9 pounds (2.7 to 4 kg) and cover 21 square feet (2 m²)! It's rare that we stop to think about our skin that way, but it's an integral part of the body. It's made up of two main layers: The outer layer is the epidermis, whose primary role is to protect the dermal tissue, which is the next layer and is made up of special cells that can sense touch, sweat and regulate body temperature.

The skin has an amazing ability to repair itself, which makes sense, since it's the front line of defense. It can tend to take a beating with scratches, cuts, windburn and sunburn, so it's important that it can be repaired quickly. However, if our immune system is compromised and we're not vibrant and healthy, the healing process of the skin will be affected.

There are things we can do to support our skin and our body's overall response to repair by drinking plenty of water, cutting down on (or cutting out) sugars and highly processed foods and making sure we're getting plenty of vegetables of all colors. There are also herbs that can be supportive to this system. Herbs such as calendula, plantain, lavender and rose are wonderfully soothing anti-inflammatory plants that can be used for a host of topical applications. In this chapter, you'll find recipes that can be used for cuts, scratches and burns. You'll also find recipes that are fabulous for cleansing, moisturizing and softening the skin. I even include a hair rinse!

DEM MUSCLES

In my early thirties, I studied holistic massage therapy. I wanted to gain a deeper understanding of the body, how it worked and how I could better use herbs to support the musculoskeletal system.

Just under the skin are three layers of muscles: superficial muscles, which lie just under the skin, with intermediate and deeper muscles underneath. Helping to keep it all together are tendons, which are a thicker tissue that attaches the muscle to bone, and ligaments, which attach bone to bone. These tendons and ligaments are what make up our joints.

Our muscles and joint tissues are amazing and need just as much love and support as the rest of our bodies. Making sure we get plenty of gentle movement daily is an important way to keep our muscles and joints engaged and active. Walking and some gentle stretching or yoga are the perfect way to give our muscles some love and attention. Creating the time for massage, whether it be self-massage or seeing a trained licensed massage therapist, is a great way to support not only the musculoskeletal system but also the digestive, lymphatic and immune systems.

Even with all the love our muscles and joint tissue receive, they can get sore and cramped, so make sure you're getting enough magnesium, calcium, potassium and B vitamins in your diet. You'll also need some handy herbal preparations that include St. John's wort, ginger and meadowsweet for when your muscles and joints need some extra TLC.

DEALING WITH PAIN

When we are feeling pain in our muscles we don't immediately think about our nervous system, but we should. Our nerves run throughout our entire body, sending information to our brain, such as pain signals. Whether we are dealing with either acute or chronic pain, it's always good to add herbs that also support the nervous system.

St. John's wort is often referred to as the depression herb, but I use it for nerve pain. I use it both topically as an infused oil and internally as a tincture. I also like to use turmeric, which is a wonderful anti-inflammatory. When we feel pain there is often some inflammation involved. So using herbs such as turmeric and ginger, especially together, can help reduce inflammation in the body, which will help reduce the pain. Other herbs, such as rose, lavender and chamomile, can also soothe the nervous system, decrease inflammation and bring some relief.

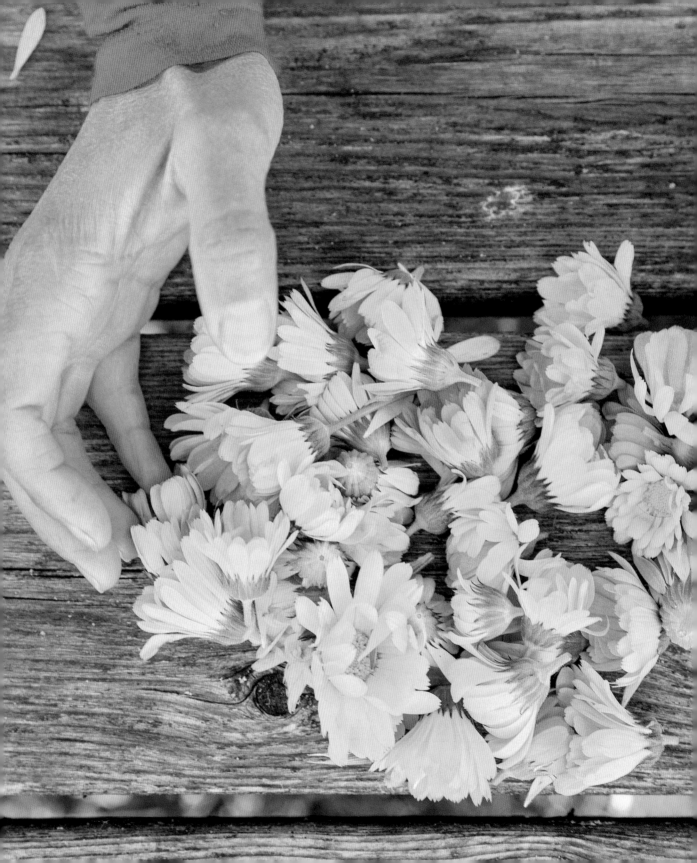

CALENDULA OIL

Makes 2 cups (480 ml)

The farm in the summer is filled with beautiful plant life and rows and rows of orange and yellow buzzing with the sounds of pollinators. Calendula is an easy plant to grow and easily self-seeds year after year. Its sticky, resinous blossoms are one of my favorite topical plants to grow and have on hand year-round. These beautiful yellow blossoms are antimicrobial, astringent, antiseptic and anti-inflammatory. They have an amazing ability to regenerate skin cells and heal wounds without scars. You can use calendula oil alone on cuts, scratches, burns and rashes or you could make the oil into dreamy Whipped Calendula Body Butter (page 152).

INGREDIENTS
2 cups (40 g) dried calendula

2 cups (480 ml) extra virgin olive oil

WHAT YOU'LL NEED
Spice grinder

16-oz (480-ml) jar

Wooden skewer or chopstick

Veggie tray heating mat (optional)

Strainer

16-oz (480-ml) jar, for storage

Run the calendula through a spice grinder, and then place it into a 16-ounce (480-ml) jar. If you don't have a grinder, you can just place the calendula into the jar. Next, slowly pour the olive oil into the jar, filling it all the way up. Then with the skewer or chopstick, push down inside the sides of the jar. You'll notice air bubbles as the oil makes its way through the calendula. As more air bubbles come up, the volume of the oil will go down. Top off the jar with oil and repeat the process with the stick. Do this a couple of times. Then place the lid on the jar. Shake and place the jar upside down for a few minutes. Shake again. Open it back up and see if there is more room to add more oil; if so, top it off.

Place the jar on a veggie tray heating mat (such as the kind used for gardening) for 1 to 2 weeks, or let the jar hang out at room temperature for 4 to 6 weeks. Once ready, strain and store in a clean 16-ounce (480-ml) jar.

TO USE
You can use the oil as it is, by rubbing onto your skin and massaging it in. Or you can make it into luscious body butters (such as the one on page 152) and healing salves (see page 155 for a method to make salve).

Note: It's best to use calendula that was harvested and dried within the year. When purchasing dried calendula, the blossoms should look bright and vibrant.

WHIPPED CALENDULA BODY BUTTER

Makes 8 oz (227 g)

I used to make a lot of lotions when I started making body products, but when I became a massage therapist, I switched over to making body butters. I preferred the creamy, light texture and richness of a whipped body butter, and because it doesn't have a water element, it's more shelf stable.

Body butters can be made out of any infused oils, and this recipe uses calendula oil. Calendula is anti-inflammatory and soothing, making this thick and luscious butter wonderful for dry, cracked skin and rashes. To make this body butter, you first need to make the Calendula Oil on page 151.

INGREDIENTS
½ oz (14 g) cocoa butter

2 oz (56 g) shea butter

3 oz (85 g) Calendula Oil (page 151)

1 tsp rose hip oil

1 tsp vitamin E oil

WHAT YOU'LL NEED
Digital scale

Small pan

Strainer

Hand mixer

4 (2-oz [60-ml]) or 8 (1-oz [30-ml]) jars, for storage

Using the scale, weigh out the cocoa butter and shea butter and melt in a small pan over low heat.

Place the oils in a bowl. Once the butters have melted, pour through a strainer into the bowl. Use a hand mixer to blend the ingredients together. Start slowly on low speed and work your way up to high speed, and whip for 1 to 2 minutes. Then place the bowl into the freezer for about 10 minutes.

Take the bowl out of the freezer and scrape down the sides with a spatula. Then mix again with the mixer, again starting on low speed and working your way up to high speed. Mix for about 1 minute. If the cream is still liquid or really soft, put the bowl back in the freezer for 5 minutes. Take it out again, then scrape and mix. If still a liquid, place back in the freezer for another 5 minutes.

Repeat this process until you have a nice whipped cream consistency. If the cream ends up in the freezer for too long, it will become too hard. So, what you can do then is slowly drizzle in more calendula oil as you whip it with the mixer. Keep adding until you achieve the consistency you like. Scoop the mixture into four 2-ounce (60-ml) or eight 1-ounce (30-ml) containers. The body butter can be stored at room temperature, out of direct heat or sunlight.

TO USE
This body butter is lovely to use on any rough or dry skin and rashes. Take a small pea-size amount and gently rub into the skin. Use as often as needed.

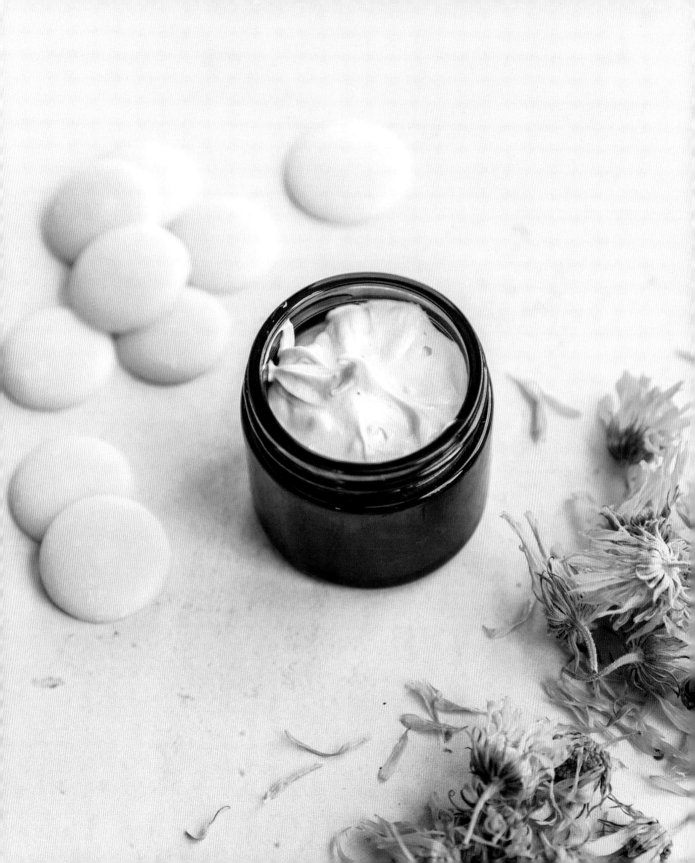

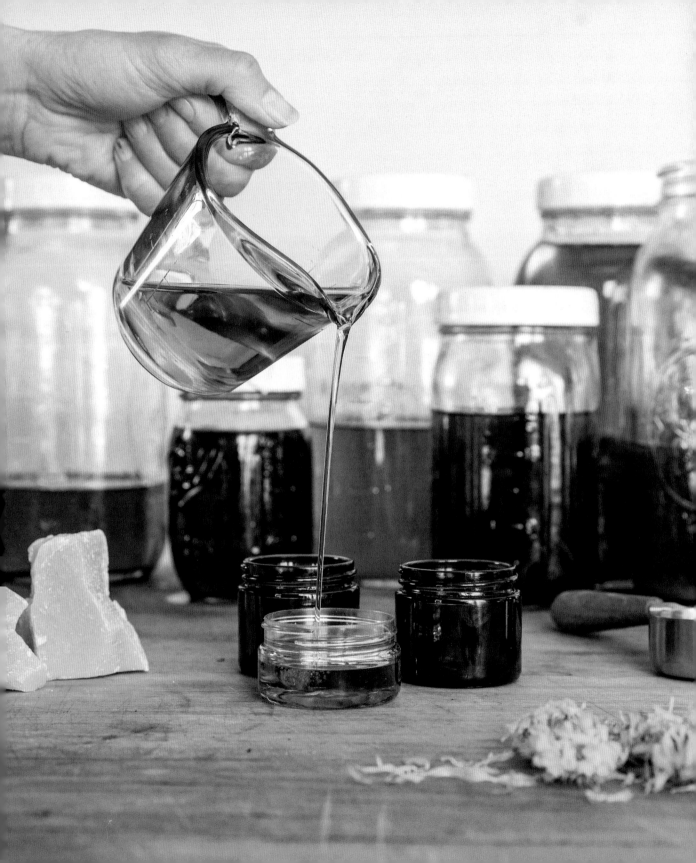

HERBAL HEALING SALVE

Makes 8 oz (227 g)

Everyone, in my opinion, should know how to make a healing salve and have an herbal healing salve handy at all times. Healing salves are made using herbs that are fabulous for healing trauma to the skin, such as cuts, bruises, bites, scratches and wounds. When I was a kid, the go-to first aid for skin was a petroleum-based product—yuck! I will stick with this blend any day over a petroleum-based one.

So, the first thing you'll need to do is make the oils. I make all these oils individually, so they are always on hand. To make all the oils, follow the same method as the Calendula Oil recipe on page 151. If you don't want to make a pint (480 ml) of oil like that recipe indicates, you can halve the recipe and make it in jam jars, or double the recipe and make into a quart (1 L)!

INGREDIENTS

¼ cup (60 ml) plantain oil

¼ cup (60 ml) Calendula Oil (page 151)

2 tbsp (30 ml) comfrey oil

2 tbsp (30 ml) St. John's wort oil, store-bought or made using only the fresh plant (see Note)

¼ cup (60 ml) yarrow oil

1–1½ oz (28–42 g) beeswax

1 tsp vitamin E oil

WHAT YOU'LL NEED

Scale

Small pan

Glass measuring cup with pour spout

4 (2-oz [60-ml]) jars or
8 (1-oz [30-ml]) jars, for storage

Make each of the herb oils individually, following the method for Calendula Oil on page 151. Once the oils are infused and strained, you can begin this salve.

Measure all the oils into a bowl. Using the scale, weigh out the beeswax, then melt it in a small pan over low heat. Once the beeswax is melted, turn off the heat. Take the bowl with all the herbal oils, pour that into the pan with beeswax and use a spoon to mix it all together.

Before pouring into the jars I like to test how hard the salve is. Take the mixture and pour a drop or two onto a piece of parchment paper or plate. Wait until it's totally cooled and solidified. If you find that it's softer than you'd like, then slowly add a little more beeswax to the blend and warm it on the stove again to melt and mix it in. If the salve is too hard, then you can add a little more oil. While you're testing the salve out, the beeswax and oil blend will most likely start to solidify. If this happens, just gently warm it back up to a liquid.

Pour the liquid into the glass measuring cup with a spout, then pour directly into your jars. As you're doing this the liquid in the pan might start to cool and solidify. If this happens, use a spatula to scrape it down, and you may need to reheat it back to liquid if it solidifies too much.

TO USE

Apply a small amount of the salve on cuts, scrapes, bruises, rashes and cracked skin. Use as often as needed. Do not use this salve on open wounds.

Note: St. John's wort medicine is most effective when made with the fresh herb, not dried. You can purchase fresh oil from a local herbalist or an herb shop. Or if you want to make it yourself, you can grow some plants and harvest them once they start to bloom. Gather a mix of flowers and buds. I do not recommend harvesting this plant wild, unless you have been trained in wild gathering. It's also important to leave some in your garden to go to seed. Fill a jar with the fresh flowers and buds, and then cover completely with olive oil and let the jar sit in the sun for 4 to 6 weeks. Since this oil is made using fresh flowers, there is a higher chance for it to mold, so it's important to check on your oil daily, making sure to add more oil to the jar, keeping all the plant material well covered.

DON'T JUST GRIN + BEAR IT TINCTURE

Makes 6–8 oz (180–240 ml)

INGREDIENTS

3 tbsp (27 g) dried turmeric powder

2 tbsp (6 g) dried German chamomile

1 tbsp (9 g) dried hawthorn berries

1 tbsp (4 g) dried California poppy

1 tsp dried ginger pieces

2 tbsp (30 ml) fresh milky oat tincture
or 3 tbsp (4 g) fresh milky oat tops
(optional, see Note)

1 tbsp (20 g) honey (optional)

About 1 cup (240 ml) vodka

WHAT YOU'LL NEED

Spice grinder

8-oz (240-ml) jar

Strainer

4 (2-oz [60-ml]) dropper bottles
or a jar, for storage

How often do you just grin and bear it, when it comes to dealing with pain? The majority of people in the world exist with some sort of daily chronic pain. Though I think it's amazing how adaptable, tolerant and resilient people are when dealing with pain, there comes a time where enough is enough.

There are a number of pain management therapies that I like to use, such as acupuncture, massage therapy, yoga/gentle stretching and, of course, herbs. When working with herbs for pain, I tend to use herbs both topically and internally that have anti-inflammatory, analgesic and antispasmodic properties and that support the nervous system and the musculoskeletal system, such as turmeric, chamomile and California poppy. Turmeric is a wonderful anti-inflammatory and I have found with regular use that it has decreased my daily knee pain. Chamomile is also a mild analgesic and anti-inflammatory, and California poppy is an antispasmodic and analgesic.

When making medicine, holding intent and vision is an important part of the process. As you're gathering your herbs, meditate on why you're making this tincture, whether it's for yourself, a family member or a friend in need. Hold your reasons for making this medicine close to you while going through the following steps.

Gather your herbs and one by one measure them out and run them through a spice grinder, then place into an 8-ounce (240-ml) jar. If you don't have a grinder, you can just measure out the herbs and place directly into the jar. If using the fresh milky oat tincture and honey, you can add them now.

Next, pour in the vodka until the jar is filled. Mix it all together and add more alcohol if needed, then place the cap on and shake. Open the jar back up and check to see if the alcohol level has dropped. If it has, add more to the jar and cover back up.

Label your jar and let sit for 4 weeks. Store in a place where you'll see it often. Shake it every week and taste a drop or two. After 4 weeks, strain and bottle in labeled 2-ounce (60-ml) dropper bottles or a jar.

TO USE

Take 1 full dropper (¼ teaspoon) one to three times a day, in water or tea, for chronic pain.

Note: This blend will be most effective using fresh milky oat tops. If you aren't able to source them fresh, you can purchase prepared fresh milky oat tincture from an herbal shop and use 1 ounce (30 ml) in this blend. Dried milky oat tops make a lovely infusion, but they don't come close to comparing to the medicinal activity of fresh milky oat tops when making a tincture. You can use an equal amount of dried, just be aware the tincture may not be as effective.

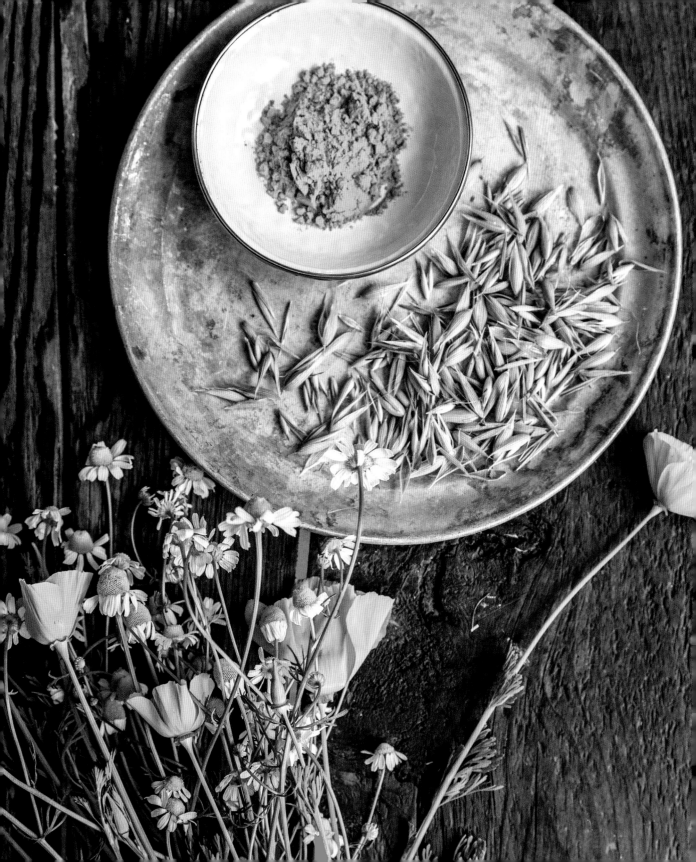

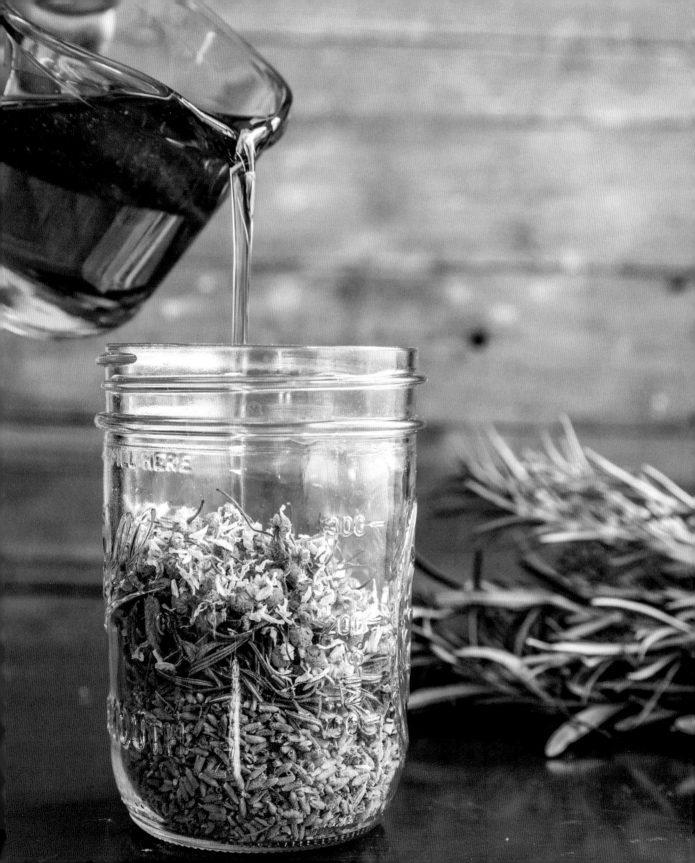

MUSCLE TENSION RELEASE OIL

Makes 16 oz (480 ml)

We work our muscles daily, even if it doesn't always feel like we do. While writing this book, I've had to slow down and spend more time seated at the computer. When I see my massage therapist, we notice how tense and tight the muscles all around my chest, shoulders and neck are because of this computer work, yet I feel like I'm barely moving. On the flip side, when farming, it's go, go, go. My body is always in motion, and often throughout the day there is something heavy involved. When I see my massage therapist in the farming months, we notice all sorts of tight and tense areas. So, whether your body is in constant movement or you work a desk job, your muscles either way will most likely experience tension. This oil, made with rosemary, meadowsweet and lavender, is a wonderful way to support muscle tissue.

Rosemary, meadowsweet and lavender are all anti-inflammatory herbs. Rosemary helps promote blood flow and circulation and decrease pain. Meadowsweet can help reduce pain, and lavender is great for relieving muscle tension and stress.

INGREDIENTS

3 tbsp (7 g) dried peppermint

3 tbsp (7 g) dried meadowsweet

3 tbsp (6 g) dried rosemary

2 tbsp (4 g) dried lavender

2 tbsp (4 g) dried chamomile

2 cups (480 ml) extra virgin olive oil

WHAT YOU'LL NEED

Spice grinder

16-oz (480-ml) jar

Wooden skewer or chopstick

Veggie tray heating mat (optional)

Strainer

16-oz (480-ml) jar, for storage

Gather the ingredients and one by one run the herbs through a spice grinder. Then, place them into a 16-ounce (480-ml) jar. If you don't have a grinder, you can just place them right into the jar.

Next, slowly pour the olive oil into the jar, filling it all the way up. With the skewer or chopstick, push down inside the sides of the jar. You'll notice air bubbles as the oil makes its way through the herbs. As more air bubbles come up, the volume of the oil will go down. So, top off the jar with oil and repeat the process with the stick. Do this a couple of times. Then place the lid on the jar. Shake and place the jar upside down for a few minutes. Shake again. Open it back up and see if there is more room to add more oil; if so, top it off.

Place the jar on a veggie tray heating mat (such as the kind used for gardening) for 1 to 2 weeks, or let the jar hang out at room temperature for 4 to 6 weeks. Once ready, strain and store in a clean 16-ounce (480-ml) jar.

TO USE

From here you can do a number of things. You can use the oil on its own and gently massage into tense, tight or sore muscles. You can also make it into a salve, following the recipe for the healing salve on page 155. If you prefer a cream, you can follow the instructions for the calendula body butter (page 152), substituting this oil for the calendula oil. To work a little deeper, you can put the oil, salve or body butter on your sore muscles, and then place a warming blanket, heating pad or hot water bottle on the muscles as well.

JOINT + TENDON OIL

Makes 16 oz (480 ml)

We have more than three hundred joints in the body, and these are made of ligaments. Ligaments are a dense connective tissue that connects bone to bone, such as our knees, elbows, ankles, hips and shoulders. Ligament tissue is thick and has far less blood flow than our muscles and other tissues do. This is one of the reasons things such as ankle sprains can take so long to heal, due to the lack of blood flow to the joint. It may also be one of the reasons joints can often feel cold.

Tendons are another dense tissue in our body that connect muscle to bone. Like ligaments, tendons are made of thick connective tissue and lack an abundance of blood flow. So, it's nice to massage these areas of the body with a warming oil that is infused with herbs such as ginger, cinnamon and rosemary, which help support circulation and stimulate blood flow. These herbs are also anti-inflammatory and help decrease pain.

I use sesame oil to make this because sesame oil is a rich and more specifically warming oil, making it a better choice for working with joints. If you don't have access to sesame oil, then I suggest using extra virgin olive oil.

INGREDIENTS

3 tbsp (20 g) dried ginger pieces

3 tbsp (6 g) dried rosemary

2 tbsp (20 g) dried cinnamon chips

2 tbsp (4 g) dried yarrow

1 tbsp (2 g) dried comfrey

2 cups (480 ml) sesame oil or extra virgin olive oil

WHAT YOU'LL NEED

Spice grinder

16-oz (480-ml) jar

Wooden skewer or chopstick

Veggie tray heating mat (optional)

Strainer

16-oz (480-ml) jar, for storage

Gather the ingredients and run the herbs one by one through the grinder. Then place them into a 16-ounce (480-ml) jar. If you don't have a grinder, you can just place them right into the jar.

Next, slowly pour the sesame oil into the jar, filling it all the way up. Then with a skewer or chopstick, push down inside the sides of the jar. You'll notice air bubbles as the oil makes its way through the herbs. As more air bubbles come up, the volume of the oil will go down. So, top off the jar with oil and repeat the process with the stick. Do this a couple of times. Then place the lid on the jar. Shake and place the jar upside down for a few minutes. Shake again. Open it back up and see if there is more room to add more oil; if so, top it off.

Place the jar on a veggie tray heating mat (such as the kind used for gardening) for 1 to 2 weeks, or let the jar hang out at room temperature for 4 to 6 weeks. Once ready, strain and store in a clean 16-ounce (480-ml) jar.

TO USE

From here you can use the oil on its own and gently massage into cold or aching joints and tendons. You can also make it into a salve, following the recipe on page 155, or if you prefer a cream-like consistency you can follow the instructions for the calendula body butter (page 152), substituting this oil for the calendula oil.

You can use the oil, salve or body butter on your joints and tendons. To work a little deeper, you can put it on and then place a warming blanket, heating pad or hot water bottle on the area as well.

Be aware that the ginger and cinnamon infused into the oil may create a warming effect on the skin—this is normal and a beneficial part of the restorative process. You may want to test a small portion of the oil on your skin for any reactions. If you find your skin is sensitive to the oil, you can dilute it with more sesame oil or olive oil to the level that works for you, or make a new batch leaving out the ginger and cinnamon.

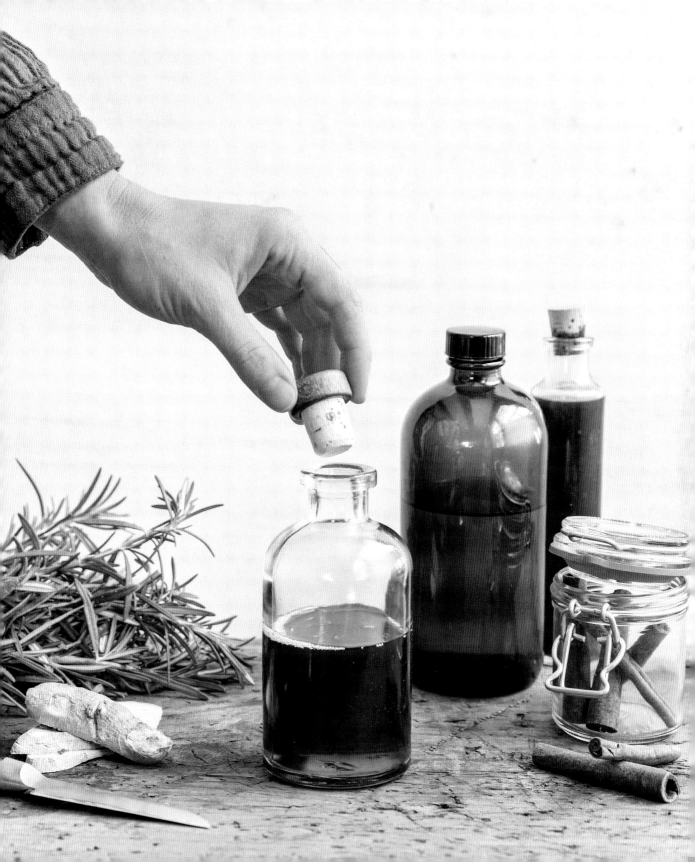

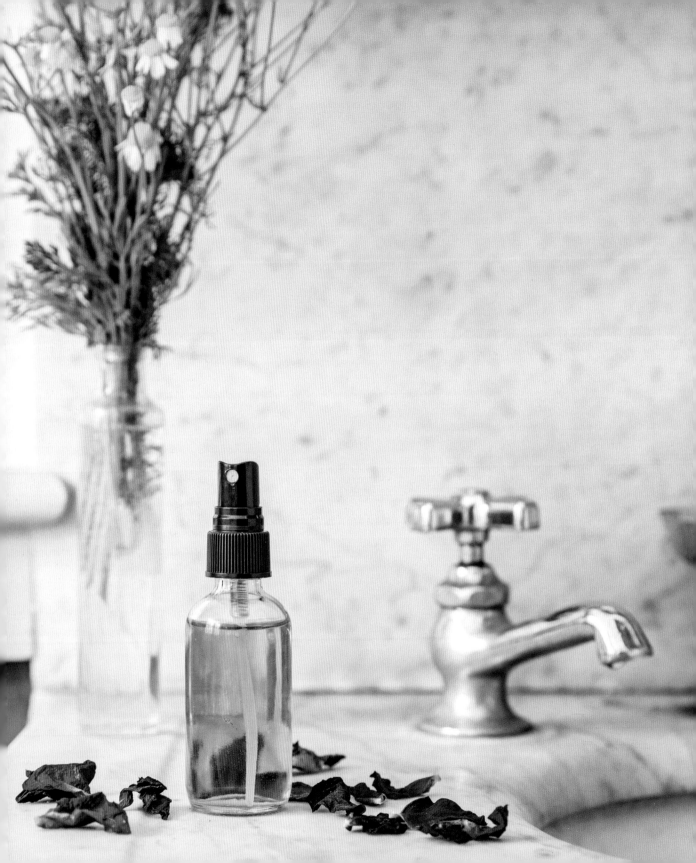

HERBAL FACIAL TONER

Makes roughly 2⅓ cups (550 ml)

There's an overwhelming amount of products on the market targeting beautiful, youthful skin, and many of these products cost a pretty penny. A great deal of these products also are made with unrecognizable ingredients that can be harmful to our bodies and the environment. I've been making my own body products for more than 20 years, and you can too! There are so many ways to utilize the soothing and cleansing properties of herbs, and this facial toner is a great place to start.

There are two versions to choose from. The Elderflower + Rose toner is a more floral scent. These herbs are both anti-inflammatory and very soothing to the skin and work well on all skin types. The Rosemary + Mint toner is invigorating and helps stimulate circulation. The addition of lemon essential oil offers a bright, uplifting scent and astringency. This is a good blend for all skin types, including acne-prone skin. Both blends are made with herbs that help with skin inflammation and puffiness.

ELDERFLOWER + ROSE

½ cup (60 g) dried elderflower

¼ cup (4 g) dried rose petals

½ tsp dried hibiscus flowers

⅓ cup (80 g) aloe gel

2 cups (480 ml) witch hazel

ROSEMARY + MINT

½ cup (6 g) dried peppermint

¼ cup (14 g) dried rosemary

⅓ cup (80 g) aloe gel

2 cups (480 ml) witch hazel

4–6 drops lemon essential oil (optional)

WHAT YOU'LL NEED

Blender (optional)

1-qt (1-L) jar

Strainer

2–4 spray bottles or decorative bottles, for storage

Gather all your herbs for the toner of your choice. Place the herbs into a blender, along with the aloe and witch hazel. Blend for about 30 seconds, just enough to incorporate the herbs, aloe and witch hazel. After it's all blended, pour into a 1-quart (1-L) jar. If you don't have a blender, you can place all the ingredients into the jar and shake the jar vigorously, until everything is well incorporated.

Cover the jar and let sit for 4 weeks. Make sure to check on it and shake the jar over the 4 weeks. After 4 weeks, you can strain the herbs from the jar. If you are making the Rosemary + Mint toner and want to add the lemon essential oil, you can do that now. Then bottle into spray bottles or decorative bottles.

TO USE

If bottled in a spray bottle, you can spray the toner on your face and body after washing or a shower. If using a bottle without a spray nozzle, you can place the toner onto a cotton pad and gently massage onto the face. Or you can place a little in your hands and splash or pat it gently onto your skin.

To create a full herbal skin care routine, start by cleaning your face with warm water and using the herbal scrub or mask on page 164. Follow it with this toner. The richness from the scrub and soothing properties of the aloe in this toner mean you shouldn't need to follow with another moisturizer, but you may use one of the herbal oils or the body butter in this chapter if you'd like.

FEED YOUR FACE HERBAL SCRUB + MASK

Makes about 2 cups (200 g)

Who doesn't want super soft skin? This blend is awesome and leaves your face feeling so soft and smooth. Our facial skin is sensitive, and it's important to use products that are gentle and supporting to the face. The herbs in this blend—lavender, rose and calendula—are all anti-inflammatory, which is perfect for soothing inflamed skin. They're also antimicrobial, astringent and gentle enough that the scrub won't strip your face of oils. This blend can be used daily as a face scrub or can be made into a face mask. It is good for all skin types.

SCRUB

1 cup (128 g) oats (quick-cooking or old-fashioned oats)

¼ cup (42 g) flax seeds

2 tbsp (4 g) dried lavender

4 tbsp (5 g) dried calendula

4 tbsp (5 g) dried rose petals

3 tbsp (18 g) nutritional yeast (optional, for acne)

MASK

Raw apple cider vinegar or lemon juice (for oily skin)

Yogurt and honey (for dry skin)

WHAT YOU'LL NEED

Spice grinder

Strainer

16-oz (480-ml) jar, for storage

TO MAKE THE SCRUB

Gather the herbs, then one by one grind each of the ingredients into a powder or fine meal. As they're ready, place them into a bowl. For the oats, after grinding you can run them through a sifter or strainer to weed out the larger pieces that didn't grind down. Mix everything together until well blended. Store in a 16-ounce (480-ml) jar or in any lovely decorative jar.

TO USE THE SCRUB

Gently wet your face, place a small amount of the scrub in your hand and add a little water. Mix in your hand to create a paste and gently massage onto your face and neck. Rinse off. Follow with the Herbal Facial Toner on page 163 and then your favorite moisturizer or cream, if you'd like.

TO MAKE THE MASK

For both options below, start with a clean, dry face.

If you have oily skin, place about 1 teaspoon of the herb/oat mixture into your palm or a small bowl. Add 1 teaspoon of a blend of raw apple cider vinegar and water until a thick paste forms (see Note).

If you have dry skin, mix about 1 teaspoon of the herb/oat mixture with a little water, yogurt and honey until a thick paste forms (see Note).

TO USE THE MASK

Massage onto your skin and leave until dry, 5 to 10 minutes. Rinse off and follow with the Herbal Facial Toner (page 163) and then your favorite moisturizer or cream, if you'd like.

Note: The exact ratio of apple cider vinegar (or yogurt and honey) to water doesn't matter; the main goal is to dilute the vinegar a little and have just enough liquid to form a paste. If you find the vinegar too drying for your skin, use less or even no vinegar next time.

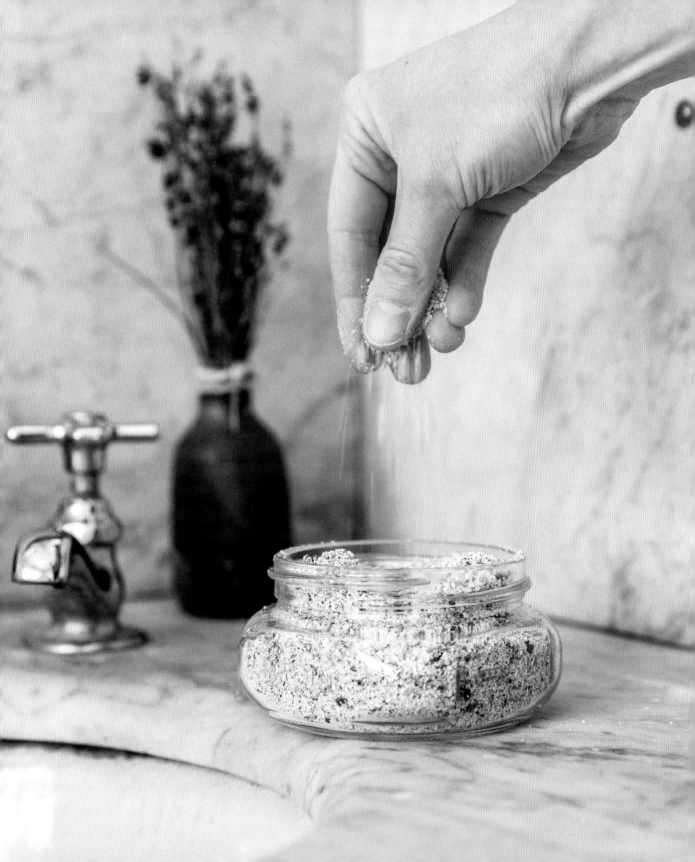

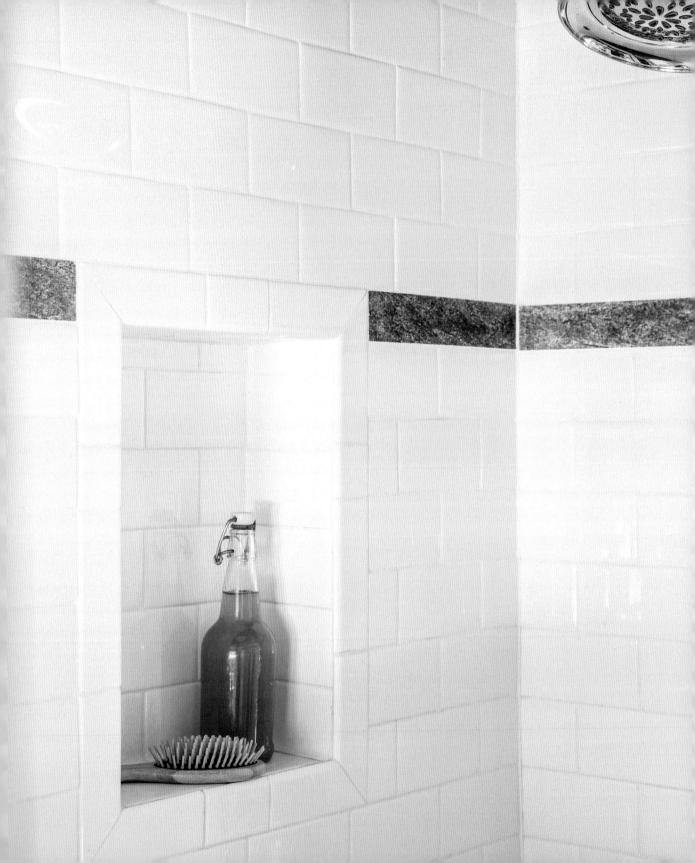

HERBAL HAIR RINSE

Makes 4 cups (960 ml) concentrate

When I was in my early twenties, I came across a fancy hair rinse at my local co-op. My hair was pretty fried from years of swimming in a pool. The hair rinse was diluted apple cider vinegar and herbs, and I loved it. It made my hair smell so nice and gave it a lovely shine. This homemade rinse gives the same effect at a fraction of the cost. It will smell like vinegar, but it will also smell like the herbs you put in it. Don't worry, the vinegar smell does not stay in your hair after it's rinsed out. I use apple cider vinegar because it is a great pH balancer. It won't strip the hair of natural oils, but it also won't coat and weigh the hair down either like conditioners can. The herbs in this blend—rosemary, nettles and kelp—are stimulating and encourage blood flow to the scalp, which promotes healthy scalp and hair growth. There are two versions below, one for dark hair and one for light hair.

HAIR RINSE BASE
¼ cup (12 g) dried nettle

2 tbsp (4 g) dried rosemary

2 tsp (7 g) dried kelp powder

2 tbsp (4 g) dried horsetail

4 cups (960 ml) raw apple cider vinegar

DARK HAIR ADDITIONS
2 tbsp (4 g) dried sage

2 tbsp (22 g) dried burdock root

2–3 drops rosemary essential oil (optional)

2–3 drops sage essential oil (optional)

2–3 drops lavender essential oil (optional)

LIGHT HAIR ADDITIONS
⅓ cup (12 g) dried chamomile

2 tbsp (4 g) dried lavender

¼ cup (6 g) dried oat straw or milky oat tops

⅓ cup (6 g) dried calendula

2–3 drops lemon essential oil (optional)

2–3 drops lavender essential oil (optional)

WHAT YOU'LL NEED
Spice grinder

1-qt (1-L) jar

Strainer

1-qt (1-L) jar, for storage

8-oz (240-ml) shower-safe bottle for making single uses of vinegar rinse

Gather all your herbs and ingredients. Measure out each of the herbs and one by one run them through a spice grinder. Then place them into the 1-quart (1-L) jar. If you don't have a grinder, you can just place them right into the jar.

Fill the jar with raw apple cider vinegar, cover and mix or shake well to ensure the herbs are submerged completely. Let the herbal mixture sit for 4 to 6 weeks. Shake and check on it regularly. After 4 to 6 weeks, you can strain the infused vinegar into a clean jar. Store the vinegar on a shelf in your bathroom for up to a year.

TO USE
Add 1 to 2 tablespoons (15 to 30 ml) of hair rinse to a shower-safe bottle, then add 1 cup (240 ml) of water to the bottle. Shake and it's ready to use. You can use it in the shower in place of conditioner or after you condition. I like to pour it right onto my scalp, massaging my scalp and pulling it through my hair down to the ends. Leave on for a minute or two while finishing up your shower, then rinse it out.

Once the herbal vinegar concentrate is mixed with water it will last for 2 to 3 weeks.

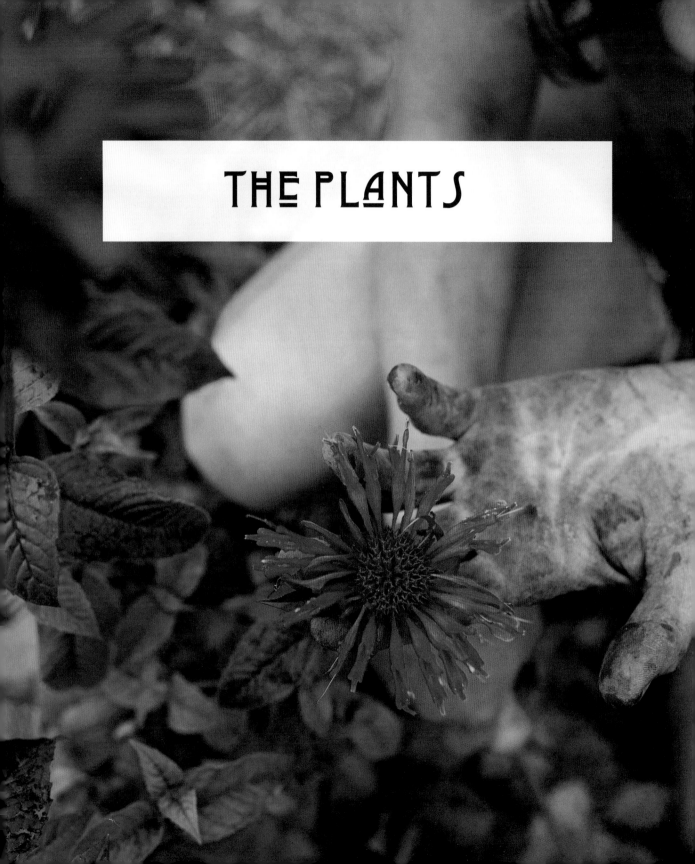

THE PLANTS

ASHWAGANDHA

Withania somnifera

Family: Solanaceae
Part used: Root
Energetics: Warming, sweet
Actions: Anti-inflammatory, aphrodisiac, nervine, immune amphoteric, reproductive tonic, sedative (mild)

Ashwagandha, native to India, grows on our farm in Maine as an annual. I harvest the roots every fall to make into tinctures and dry for teas, soup stocks and powder. Ashwagandha is a wonderful adaptogen that can be used as a daily tonic. It is part of the nightshade family, so if you have allergies you may want to avoid this herb. Otherwise, it's a wonderfully rejuvenating and nourishing herb that I like to use as a brain tonic and to clear up brain fog and poor memory. It helps induce sleep, relieves anxiety and stress and is great for supporting the reproductive system. Ashwagandha is a great herb for rebuilding vitality and overall strength in the body.

Contraindications: Avoid use if allergic to nightshades or if you have hyperthyroidism or elevated iron levels.

ASTRAGALUS

Astragalus membranaceus

Family: Fabaceae/Leguminosae
Part used: Root
Energetics: Sweet, warming, moist
Actions: Anti-inflammatory, antioxidant, cardiotonic, immune amphoteric, nutritive tonic

Astragalus, part of the pea family, is a perennial that we grow here on the farm. We harvest the roots in its third year to make into tinctures or dry for teas, soup stocks, syrups and elixirs. Astragalus is a great herb to use when building back strength and vitality. I like to use it as an immune support to help prevent colds and flu and help with allergies. Astragalus is a rejuvenative herb for when you are depleted and weak, helping restore vitality and energy. Helps improve digestion, nutrient absorption and cardiovascular function. This is a great front-line herb for immune support and preventive care.

Contraindications: None known.

BLUE VERVAIN

Verbena hastata

Family: Verbenaceae
Part used: Flowers, leaves
Energetics: Bitter, acrid, cooling, drying
Actions: Antispasmodic, anxiolytic, bitter, diaphoretic, emmenagogue, expectorant, nervine

Blue vervain is a great herb to add to any garden. When we moved to the farm, I found a couple of plants growing wild along the stream. I loved that so much. I like to use blue vervain for nervous system issues such as anxiety, especially associated with PMS and menopause, and it can also be used for spasms and tics. As a diaphoretic, it's been used for relieving fevers and other flu symptoms, such as aching muscles, and could be an addition for the Fever Break Tea on page 66 or a replacement for boneset.

Contraindications: Avoid use during pregnancy; excessive use may cause nausea.

BURDOCK

Arctium lappa

Family: Asteraceae/Compositae
Part used: Roots, seeds, leaves
Energetics: Sweet, salty, cooling, moist
Actions: Alterative, anti-inflammatory, antioxidant, demulcent, hepatoprotective (mild), lymph tonic

Burdock is a weed that everyone should know and love. I mostly use the roots and will harvest them in the spring and fall to eat fresh, tincture and dry for tea, soup stocks and syrups. I love using this herb for clearing toxins from the gut, supporting elimination and purifying the blood. I like to use it for inflamed skin conditions that are hot and red, such as acne, rosacea, rashes, etc. Burdock is a pre/probiotic and helps support healthy flora in the digestive tract.

Contraindications: None known.

CALENDULA

Calendula officinalis

Family: Asteraceae/Compositae
Part used: Flowers
Energetics: Cooling, bitter, pungent
Actions: Alterative, anti-inflammatory, antioxidant, antiviral, astringent, immunostimulant, lymph tonic

Calendula is such a beautiful little ray of sunshine. We grow rows and rows of this wonderful herb and harvest its blossoms well into the fall. We make it into a fresh tincture and dry it for teas, soup stock and oil. Externally, I like to use calendula on hot, irritated skin conditions, and it's my top go-to herb for rashes, cuts and abrasions. I love adding this to soup stocks in the wintertime and other immune teas or baths. I add it to teas for soothing the intestinal tract and gut and to support digestion and absorption. I regularly use this herb for any congestion related to the lymphatic system, such as swollen glands, and it makes a great mouthwash for gum inflammation.

Contraindications: None known.

CALIFORNIA POPPY

Eschscholzia californica

Family: Papaveracea
Part used: Root, flower, leaf
Energetics: Cooling, bitter
Actions: Analgesic, antispasmodic, anxiolytic, nervine, sedative

California poppy is a plant that I swoon over. Every year I try to grow the California poppy patch on the farm to get bigger and bigger. I harvest the entire plant throughout the growing season as it flowers and tincture the entire plant fresh. This is a wonderful herb that I like to use for pain relief, sleep issues and anxiety.

Contraindications: None known.

CATNIP

Nepeta cataria

Family: Lamiaceae/Labiate
Part used: Leaves, flowering tops
Energetics: Spicy, pungent, warming, neutral
Actions: Antispasmodic, carminative, diaphoretic, nervine, sedative (mild)

Catnip is a must on this farm. We have four, and not just to keep our four farm cats happy. Their names are Skeletor, Battlecat, Covergirl and Megababy, and they'd for sure revolt if we were to ever stop growing this tasty mint. I love using this herb for colds, flus and especially in children's formulas. I like to add it to formulas for anxiety, sleep issues, tension headaches, PMS and menstrual cramps for its medicinal properties, and for its mild mint taste. It can also be helpful for stress-related digestive issues. Catnip is easy to grow from seed and transplants. I harvest the leaves and flowers throughout the growing season to dry for teas and tinctures.

Contraindications: None known.

CAYENNE

Capsicum annuum

Family: Solanaceae
Part used: Fruit
Energetics: Pungent, heating, drying
Actions: Analgesic, anti-inflammatory, antioxidant, carminative, circulatory stimulant, diaphoretic, expectorant

Cayenne can be great for increasing peripheral circulation, especially for cold hands and feet. It's helpful in preventing arteriosclerosis and lowering LDL cholesterol. I love adding a little heat to meals for boosting circulation. I add cayenne to roasted veggies, soups, salad dressings, salsas, chocolates, sauces and just about everything that profiles, flavorwise, with heat. I also like to make a warming circulatory oil with sesame or olive oil, for topical use (see page 123).

Contraindications: Avoid use with digestive issues such as IBS, GERD and SIBO and please avoid contact with any sensitive places.

CHAMOMILE (GERMAN)
Matricaria recutita

Family: Asteraceae
Part used: Flowers
Energetics: Sweet, bitter, warming
Actions: Anti-inflammatory, antispasmodic, carminative, diaphoretic, nervine

Chamomile was in abundance this year on the farm. I think I planted over a thousand plants! We harvest the blossoms well into the fall to use for tinctures, teas, oils and elixirs. It's an easy and wonderful plant to grow from seed or transplant. Spending time with this plant is sure to increase your flow of creativity and inspiration. I use this wonderful aromatic bitter for digestive issues such as cramping, bloating, gas and stress-based digestive upset. It's a great herb to use for anxiety, inflammation, menstrual cramps and sleep issues.

Contraindications: Avoid using if you have ragweed allergies.

CINNAMON
Cinnamomum verum

Family: Lauraceae
Part used: Inner bark
Energetics: Pungent, sweet, warming
Actions: Analgesic, anti-inflammatory, antioxidant, carminative, peripheral vasodilator

Cinnamon isn't a plant that grows here in Maine, but it is something that I use often. One, because I love the way it tastes and two, because it's one of those common kitchen herbs that almost everyone has on hand, I tend to use cinnamon as often as I can. I like to use cinnamon for digestive support and warming the body, helping to get the blood moving and shaking to my cold fingers and toes. I also like to use it internally for pain and cramps and externally as an oil for joint and muscle pain relief.

Contraindications: None known.

DANDELION
Taraxacum officinale

Family: Asteraceae
Part used: Root, leaves, flowers
Energetics: Bitter, sweet, cooling
Actions: Alterative (mild), bitter tonic, diuretic (mild), hepatoprotective (mild)

Dandelion is a deep love, the mascot of my business and the inspiration behind the name Herbal Revolution. It was one of the first herbs I learned to work with on a deep level. I eagerly await the arrival of spring each year, so I can see the fields on the farm turn into a sea of beautiful yellow. I harvest the roots, leaves and flowers in the spring and fall to eat, tincture and dry for tea, soup stocks, oils and vinegars. I love using dandelion for digestive and liver support, lymph congestion, especially in the breasts, and skin conditions.

Contraindications: None known.

FENNEL
Foeniculum vulgare

Family: Apiacea
Part used: Seeds
Energetics: Sweet, mildly warming, moist
Actions: Anti-inflammatory, antispasmodic, antioxidant, aromatic, carminative, diuretic

Fennel is one of my favorite remedies for relieving bloating and gas. I like to eat a pinch of fennel after a meal or anytime I start to feel a little bloated. It tends to work every time!

It also can be helpful for relieving pain and menstrual cramps, increasing breast milk and promoting perspiration.

Contraindications: None known.

GINGER

Zingiber officinale

Family: Zingiberaceae
Part used: Rhizomes
Energetics: Pungent, sweet, warming
Actions: Anti-inflammatory, antioxidant, carminative, circulatory stimulant, diaphoretic, expectorant, nootropic

Ginger is all kinds of wonderful as a circulatory herb and heart tonic. It's good for helping increase peripheral circulation, and studies are showing that ginger can lower triglycerides and blood sugar levels. Ginger is great for nausea, bloating, gas, circulation, sore throats, pain relief and so much more. I use fresh ginger liberally as a food and add it to veggies, dressings, sauces, baked goods, soups and just about everything that pairs well with its flavor. It makes a delicious tea and infuses well in honey, vinegar and alcohol. I also like to make a warming circulatory oil for topical use (see page 123).

Contraindications: None known.

HAWTHORN

Crataegus oxyacantha

Family: Rosaceae
Part used: Flowers, leaves, berries
Energetics: Sour, sweet, warming, drying
Actions: Anti-inflammatory, antioxidant, antispasmodic, astringent, cardio trophorestorative, nervine, vasodilator

Hawthorn is food for the heart. It's fabulous for supporting, nourishing and protecting the heart and circulatory system. It's also good for memory, confusion and metabolism. Part of the rose family, hawthorn is a trophorestorative for the cardiovascular system, specifically the heart and circulatory system, but it's also an important medicine for the emotional heart. I always have some form of hawthorn medicine in remedies to support a broken and wounded heart. Generally speaking, when I formulate for the heart, I'm always holding space and thinking about both the physical and the emotional heart because they often go hand in hand. I harvest the flowers in the spring to dry or make fresh into a flower essence or tincture and the berries in the fall to make into a tincture or dry for teas and syrups. This is a medicine I like to use as a food when possible and take on a regular basis.

Contraindications: Consult with your ND, MD if you are taking heart medications such as digoxin, anticoagulants, hypertension medications or depressants.

HOPS

Humulus lupulus

Family: Cannabaceae
Part used: Strobiles
Energetics: Bitter, astringent, cooling
Actions: Analgesic, anxiolytic, astringent, bitter tonic, sedative

Hops is a beautiful vining plant that is so much fun to grow and harvest. I love harvesting this plant in the late summer for our sleep formulas and teas because hops are great for sleep issues, stress and anxiety. I used to love making my own beer, and especially herbal beer. Hops are often the bitter, fruity notes that can be tasted in IPAs and other beers that are made with hops, which are great digestive bitters. Hops can be helpful when dealing with stress-induced digestive issues. You can also enjoy hops in tea blends.

Contraindications: None known.

LADY'S MANTLE

Alchemilla vulgaris

Family: Rosaceae
Part used: Leaf
Energetics: Salty, bitter, cooling, drying
Actions: Anti-inflammatory, antioxidant, astringent, styptic, uterine tonic

Lady's mantle lines the edges of our gardens. It's a magical plant and if you've ever spent time with one early in the morning before the dew has had a chance to evaporate, you'd see what I mean. The beautiful leaves hold dew or water from rain in a way that feels like alchemy is at work. And it is. We harvest the leaves and make fresh into a tincture or dry for tea. I like to use lady's mantle for the female reproductive system as a uterine tonic, to help those who experience excessive bleeding and heavy periods with cramps. It can also help treat diarrhea and urinary incontinence.

Contraindications: None known.

LAVENDER
Lavandula officinalis

Family: Lamiaceae
Part used: Flowers
Energetics: Bitter, cooling, fragrant
Actions: Analgesic (topical), antidepressant, anti-inflammatory, antioxidant, antispasmodic, anxiolytic carminative, nervine, nootropic

Lavender is an aromatic perennial that makes a gorgeous border that is well loved by the bees and other local pollinators. I harvest the flowering spikes during the summer to dry for tea, baking, elixirs, syrups, oils and herb bundles. There are so many lovely ways to work with lavender. It's a wonderful herb to use on its own or in formulas for stress-induced depression, anxiety, nervous exhaustion and headaches. I also like adding it to blends for sleep and digestive issues like gas, bloating and nervous stomach issues like IBS.

Contraindications: None known.

LEMON BALM
Melissa officinalis

Family: Lamiaceae
Part used: Leaves, flowers
Energetics: Sour, cooling, neutral
Actions: Antidepressant, antioxidant, antispasmodic, anxiolytic, antiviral, carminative, nervine

Lemon balm is an herb that we use a lot of at Herbal Revolution. This is a wonderful plant that is so fabulous for the nervous system. It can be calming, uplifting, focusing and supporting to our digestive, immune and nervous systems. It's also delicious. What's not to love? The aromatics always tend to be my favorite rows to weed on the farm, and for good reason. Lemon balm is loaded with volatile essential oils, so just being around and smelling the plant is incredibly medicinal. I use lemon balm for anxiety, stress, immune support and herpes and for uplifting the spirit and clearing the mind.

Contraindications: Theoretically, taking large amounts of lemon balm can have effects on people with hypothyroidism and taking Synthroid or other thyroid-stimulating medications.

LEMONGRASS
Cymbopogon citratus

Family: Graminaceae
Part used: Leaves, root
Energetics: Sweet, sour, cooling, drying
Actions: Antioxidant, antibacterial, carminative, diaphoretic

Lemongrass grows in lovely rows on the edges of our growing plots on the farm. Here in Maine, lemongrass is an annual, but in warmer climates it is a lovely perennial. We harvest it in the fall every year to dry for tea. I love its mild lemon flavor and use it for digestive blends, as it can help with gas, bloating and abdominal pain.

Contraindications: None known.

LICORICE
Glycyrrhiza glabra

Family: Fabaceae
Part used: Root
Energetics: Sweet, slightly bitter, moist, warming
Actions: Antihistamine, anti-inflammatory, antiviral, demulcent, expectorant, immune amphoteric

Licorice is an herb I'm trying to grow more of on the farm. We use the roots in our tea and tincture blends. Licorice is a sweet herb, almost too sweet for my taste, but I've yet to find another person who feels that way. So it's a great herb to add to formulas that you want to bring a little sweetness to. Licorice is a wonderful herb that is great for adrenal support and to soothe irritated tissue in the upper respiratory and digestive tracts.

Contraindications: Avoid if pregnant or if you have hypertension, congestive heart failure, edema, hyperkalemia or kidney disease. Avoid if you are taking digoxin, MAOIs, SSRIs, diuretics, anti-hypertensives or anticoagulants.

MAITAKE
Grifola frondosa

Family: Meripilaceae
Part used: Fruiting body, mycelium
Energetics: Sweet, warming, moist
Actions: Antibacterial, antifungal, antitumor, antiviral, hepatoprotective, immune amphoteric, immune tonic

Maitake, also known as hen of the woods, is a well-loved mushroom to wild foragers, and for good reason. It's tasty. Once you know how to identify it safely, it's an easy mushroom to find, and you can find large amounts. Once Gus came home with one that was over 40 pounds (18 kg)! I still remember that day clearly; what a find! We had some delicious meals that week and good medicine was made. I like to eat it or dry it for future use in soup stocks and double extractions, and we use it in our award-winning Elderberry Elixir, mushroom elixir and all other sorts of formulas for its immune support. Maitake is a great choice for supporting people with either compromised immune systems due to illness, disease or cancer or an overactive immune system such as autoimmune diseases. It's also protective to the liver and can help lower cholesterol.

Contraindications: Avoid if you have allergies to mushrooms.

MARSHMALLOW
Althea officinalis

Family: Malvaceae
Part used: Roots, leaves, flowers
Energetics: Sweet, bland, cooling, moist
Actions: Analgesic, anti-inflammatory, demulcent, diuretic

Marshmallow is a beautiful tall perennial that we grow a lot of here on the farm. It tends to like moist areas, and so I plant it in the parts of the garden that have a little heavier soil or drain a little slower than other areas. We harvest the leaves, flowers and roots for tinctures, and dry it for tea. It's a soothing and cooling plant to inflamed mucosal tissue in the body. So, I like to use it to soothe inflamed digestive and upper respiratory tracts. I use it in digestive tract formulas and in blends for the throat and lungs, especially for dry coughs.

Contraindications: None known.

MILKY OAT TOPS AND OATS
Avena sativa

Family: Poaceae
Part used: Fresh milky tops (immature grain)
Energetics: Sweet, moist
Actions: Antispasmodic, anxiolytic, demulcent, nervine, nervous system trophorestorative, nootropic, nutritive

Oats are often used in farming as a cover crop, and we use them on the farm regularly. For medicinal purposes, we harvest the oat tops when they're in the milky state. You squeeze the oat tops and a thick milky substance comes out. This is the good stuff. If left alone, the seed would continue to grow into an oat groat, where it would be hulled and either kept whole or processed into oats. Oats are an incredible food for our nervous and cardiovascular systems. Oats are high in beta-glucan, which helps lower cholesterol and high blood pressure, and they are high in antioxidants and are anti-inflammatory. I like to use milky oats to help reduce stress and anxiety, and to help support symptoms of withdrawal from certain drugs and cigarettes. They're also a great herb for firing up the libido!

Contraindications: None known.

MOTHERWORT
Leonurus cardiaca

Family: Lamiaceae
Part used: Leaf, flowers
Energetics: Bitter, cooling, drying
Actions: Antispasmodic, anxiolytic, cardiotonic, carminative, sedative

Motherwort, or lion heart, is part of the mint family, and is a lovely plant that is so easy to grow. I always feel the garden is well protected with the healthy stand of motherwort to overlook the garden from the edges. I harvest the young leaves and flowers through the summer for fresh tincture. This is a great medicine for anxiety, especially PMS-induced anxiety and anxiety with heart palpitations. Motherwort can be helpful for other PMS and menopausal symptoms, such as irritability, hot flashes and insomnia. When my partner, Gus, asks me if I've taken my motherwort, that's my hint that I need an attitude adjustment. I often use motherwort in heart formulas for preventing heart palpitations, reducing stress and lowering high blood pressure. I really love this plant and its medicine.

Contraindications: Avoid use if pregnant or if you have heavy or prolonged bleeding during your menstrual cycle.

NETTLE
Urtica dioica

Family: Urticaceae
Part used: Leaves, roots, seeds
Energetics: Salty, cooling, drying
Actions: Anti-inflammatory, antioxidant, astringent (mild), diuretic, nutritive

Nettles is the plant that I dream of all winter long. I eagerly wait for the snow to melt and make way for the nutrient-dense young leaves of nettles. I love eating the young leaves in the spring and harvesting the plant throughout the season to dry for tea, oils, soup stocks and vinegars. Regular use of nettles will support the adrenal system and nourish the kidneys and heart. Nettles have been known to boost energy levels and balance blood sugar levels. Nettles are also helpful with chronic skin issues, such as eczema and psoriasis, and I also like to use nettle-infused vinegar as a hair rinse.

Contraindications: Contact with the leaves may cause a rash; also use caution if taking digoxin or lithium.

PEPPERMINT
Mentha piperita

Family: Lamiaceae
Part used: Aerial parts
Energetics: Pungent, cooling, drying
Actions: Analgesic (topical), antidepressant, antiviral, antispasmodic, carminative, diaphoretic (mild)

Peppermint and other mints are easy plants to grow and have in your garden. They also make a lovely plant for container gardens. They easily spread, so keep an eye on this one, as it can get out of hand. Peppermint is such a delicious aromatic plant. I love its cooling energetics and use it to relieve nausea, cramping, gas, bloating, intestinal spasms and menstrual cramps. It makes a wonderful tea and I find it to also be uplifting.

Contraindications: None known.

RED CLOVER BLOSSOM
Trifolium pratense

Family: Fabaceae
Part used: Flowers, leaves
Energetics: Sweet, salty, cooling, moist
Actions: Alterative, demulcent, expectorant, lymphatic tonic, nutritive

Red clover is a plant that we use as a cover crop here on the farm for its ability to fix nitrogen in the soil, but it's also an incredible medicinal. We harvest the blossoms when they're beautiful and vibrant and dry them to use in tea and vinegar. I use red clover for lymphatic congestion, swollen lymph nodes, skin issues and cleansing the blood. Red clover has been used for hot flashes during menopause as well as for circulation and thinning the blood. If you live near an organic farm, you should check to see if they grow red clover as a cover crop. If they do, it's worth asking whether they'd let you harvest some of the red clover blossoms. Harvesting and drying your own means you'll have good-quality flowers throughout the winter season. You can buy it, but it tends to be expensive because it's so labor-intensive. If you do buy it, I suggest purchasing from a smaller local herb farm or Healing Spirit Farm, Zack Woods or Oshala Farm.

Contraindications: None known.

REISHI

Ganoderma lucidum, G. tsugae

Family: Ganodermataceae
Part used: Bitter, warming, neutral
Actions: Adaptogen, anti-inflammatory, antioxidant, antiviral, cardiotonic, hepatoprotective, immune amphoteric, nervine

Reishi is a polypore mushroom, and here in Maine, the beautiful fruiting body, *Ganoderma tsugae*, grows on fallen hemlock trees. It is distinctively unique from other polypores as it grows on a stem. I love using reishi for many things, including allergies and tension, as well as for immune and heart support. Reishi is a heart tonic that helps lower blood pressure, reduce pain caused by angina and may have the potential to help prevent arteriosclerosis and lower triglyceride levels, which can contribute to strokes and heart attacks. Reishi is not edible but is a wonderful medicine. In order to extract the medicinal properties from it, reishi should be cooked at a simmer for at least 4 hours, which makes it great for soup stocks. To make a tincture, you would want to first cook the mushroom and then combine the water, alcohol and the marc to macerate together for 4 weeks.

Contraindications: Avoid if you have allergies to mushrooms.

ROSE

Rosa rugosa, Rosa gallica

Family: Rosaceae
Part used: Flowers, leaves, hips
Energetics: Sweet, bitter, moist
Actions: Anti-inflammatory, antidepressant, cardiotonic (mild), nervine

Wild beach rose grows all over the Maine coast, and we grow it in abundance here on the farm. Rose has a long history of being associated with the heart, through poems, stories, tales, songs and tattoos, of course. Rose is a wonderful heart tonic and nervine, which has a supportive effect on the physical heart; I also like to use rose for its energetic effects on the heart. It can be beneficial for broken hearts, grief and depression. I harvest the flowers fresh and tincture them immediately in alcohol and honey or dry them for later use in tinctures and teas. If you don't have access to lovely wild roses, then I suggest getting dried apothecary rose petals that are organic, as these plants are heavily sprayed.

Contraindications: None known.

ROSEMARY

Rosmarinus officinalis

Family: Lamiaceae
Part used: Leaves
Energetics: Spicy, warming, drying
Actions: Anti-inflammatory, antioxidant, antiviral, carminative, cerebral stimulant, nervine, nootropic

Rosemary is an incredible herb that most everyone has in their kitchen. We grow rosemary in the hot and well-drained areas on the farm. We harvest it in the fall and dry it for tea, soup stocks, oils and honey. Rosemary is a fabulous herb to use regularly in your meals, especially in the colder months. It's warming and stimulating and has antiviral and antibacterial properties. It's also a wonderful plant for uplifting the spirit and mood. I like to use rosemary as a brain tonic and for helping with focus and mental clarity. It can be supportive in anxiety formulas and to help alleviate stagnant depression.

Contraindications: None known.

SCHISANDRA

Schisandra sinensis

Family: Magnoliaceae
Part used: Berries
Energetics: Pungent, bitter, sour, salty, sweet, warming, drying
Actions: Adaptogen, anti-inflammatory, antioxidant, astringent, hepatoprotective, immune amphoteric, nervine, nootropic

Schisandra is a great herb for supporting and protecting the liver, blood and circulation. This is a great herb for vitality, rejuvenation and increasing energy. It makes a great brain tonic, and I like to use it for clarity and concentration. This is a plant that grows in Maine. We don't have schisandra vines on the farm yet, but will this coming season! We use the berries to make tinctures, syrups and vinegars. The berries can be pretty intense in flavor. They carry all five tastes, although I'll say that I never get beyond the sour, bitter, pungent flavor.

Contraindications: May possibly cause digestive upset; avoid use if on blood-thinning medications such as Warfarin.

TULSI / HOLY BASIL / SACRED BASIL

Ocimum tenuiflorum

Family: Lamiaceae
Part used: Leaves
Energetics: Sweet, spicy, warming, neutral
Actions: Adaptogen (mild), antidepressant, antioxidant, antispasmodic, antiviral, carminative, expectorant, immune amphoteric, neuroprotective, nootropic

Tulsi, also known as sacred basil or holy basil, is a wonderful annual here in Maine. This plant is so easy to grow and a favorite for pollinators. It's a plant that I recommend everyone should grow and it grows well in containers. As with its cousin, culinary basil, you pinch the flowers to keep the plant bushing and branching out. I use the leaves and flowers all summer long to make into refreshing teas and drinks using our vinegar shrubs. Tulsi is a wonderful medicinal plant. I use it for uplifting the spirit and clearing the mind. This is a wonderful brain tonic for helping clear mental fog, bringing on clarity and focus but not in an overstimulating way. It's calming and supporting to the nervous system, and I like to use it in formulas to help relieve anxiety. It's also great for the digestive system, relieving gas and bloating, and for immune support.

Contraindications: None known.

TURMERIC

Curcuma longa

Family: Zingiberaceae
Part used: Rhizomes
Energetics: Bitter, pungent, warming, drying
Actions: Anti-inflammatory, antioxidant, antispasmodic, carminative, hepatoprotective, immunoregulator, nutritive

Turmeric is an herb that I often use. I eat it regularly. We don't grow it on the farm, but other farmers are growing it in Maine and other New England states. Eating turmeric is my number one way of using it. I add it to many foods, smoothies, cookies, soups, curries and golden milk drinks. If I'm not eating it, I like tincturing it. Turmeric is an herb that can be tough for our bodies to absorb, so it's important to add either ginger or black pepper to your formula too. I use turmeric for supporting the liver and aiding in detoxification, and it's great for digestive support and soothing the gut. I also like to use it for keeping general inflammation in the body at bay, especially in the digestive system and the joints.

Contraindications: None known.

YARROW

Achillea millefolium

Family: Asteraceae
Part used: Flowers, leaves
Energetics: Bitter, pungent, drying
Actions: Anti-inflammatory, antispasmodic, antiviral, astringent, bitter tonic, diaphoretic, hepatoprotective, styptic

Yarrow is a perennial that grows wild here in Maine and many other places as well. Before buying the farm, when we looked at it, I remember feeling so happy and safe seeing all the wild yarrow on the land. I like to use yarrow energetically in the form of flower essence, infused oil, hydrosol and as a balm for protection, keeping clear boundaries and not taking on the energies of others. We harvest the flowers and leaves throughout the summer when they're most vital and dry them for teas, oils and tinctures. This is a great herb to use at the onset of a cold or flu. Yarrow can be beneficial for people dealing with IBS, Crohn's, colitis, leaky gut and SIBO. It's useful for heavy menstrual bleeding and cramping, and I use it topically for bruises and sprains.

Contraindications: Avoid if allergic to ragweed; taking in large amounts may cause nausea and vomiting.

YELLOW DOCK

Rumex crispus

Family: Polygonaceae
Part used: Root
Energetics: Bitter, cooling, drying
Actions: Alterative, anti-inflammatory, astringent, bitter tonic, laxative (mild)

Yellow dock is one of the first herbs I worked with. I've dealt with anemia my whole life, and I remember many years ago making myself a syrup out of yellow dock. Every time I smell this root, I flash back to those younger years of exploration and experimenting. I love the taste and smell of this plant! I use it still in mineral- and iron-supporting syrups and blends. It's a great herb for the liver and digestive system, and I often use it for digestive support. It can be effective in blends for constipation or daily elimination support. Yellow dock grows wild on the farm, and we harvest the roots in the spring and fall. We dry it to use in tea blends, tonics and tinctures.

Contraindications: Avoid use if you have elevated iron levels or a history of kidney stones.

GLOSSARY OF ACTIONS

Adaptogen: helps us adapt to external and internal stresses.

Alterative: helps support normal elimination function and often used to help support the activity performed by the liver, kidneys, skin, lymph and lungs.

Analgesic: helps reduce and relieve pain.

Antidepressant: helps reduce depression.

Antihistamine: helps inhibit the effects of histamine, reducing symptoms of allergic reactions.

Anti-inflammatory: helps reduce inflammation throughout the body.

Antioxidant: helps remove damaging oxidized agents in living organisms.

Antiseptic: helps inhibit and prevent the growth of disease-causing microorganisms.

Antispasmodic: helps reduce and relieve spasms and cramps.

Anxiolytic: helps reduce anxiety.

Astringent: helps contract and reduce secretions in skin cells and other body tissue.

Antiviral: has effects against viruses.

Bitter tonic: helps promote and aid digestion and absorption; stimulates digestive secretions.

Cardiotonic: helps support the heart and circulatory system.

Carminative: helps relieve and expel intestinal gas.

Decongestant: helps relieve congestion in nasal passages.

Demulcent: helps soothe irritated tissue, often mucosal tissue.

Diaphoretic: helps promote perspiration.

Diuretic: helps eliminate water and electrolytes through the kidneys.

Emmenagogue: helps promote menstrual flow.

Expectorant: helps expel mucus from the respiratory system via the air passageways.

Hepatic: helps support and promote healthy liver function.

Hepatoprotective: helps protect the liver.

Hypotensive: helps lower blood pressure.

Immune amphoteric: helps normalize and regulate either depressed or excessive immune function.

Immunostimulant: helps stimulate the immune system.

Laxative: helps stimulate bowel function and peristalsis.

Lymphatic tonic: helps support the functions of the lymphatic system.

Mucilaginous: a viscous and gelatinous constituent in some seeds and plants.

Nervine: helps soothe and relax the nervous system.

Nootropic: helps enhance cerebral function and circulation.

Nutritive: helps nourish the body.

Probiotic: beneficial bacteria that help support the digestive system.

Reproductive tonic: helps support and nourish the reproductive organs.

Sedative: helps reduce anxiety and pain and induce sleepiness and relaxation.

Stimulant: excites or stimulates the nervous system.

Styptic: helps contract tissue, specifically for stopping bleeding by contracting blood vessels.

Trophorestorative: nourishes, tones and strengthens a specific organ or a function.

RESOURCES

The availability and accessibility of information, education and books on herbalism is immense. It's nothing like when I started. Having all this access, though, can also be daunting. With everyone online making claims about this and that, it can sometimes be challenging to weed out who knows what. In this list, I share my tried-and-true herbal book recommendations along with my favorite herbalists, herbal product brands, podcasts and more! Please check out Herbal Revolution Farm and Apothecary for online courses, on-site education and purchasing herbs, herbal products and more.

FIELD GUIDES

National Audubon Society Field Guide to North American Mushrooms (National Audubon Society Field Guides)

Edible Wild Plants, by Lee Peterson

Peterson Field Guide to Medicinal Plants and Herbs of Eastern and Central North America, 3rd ed., by Steven Foster and James Duke

Peterson Field Guide to Western Medicinal Plants and Herbs, by Christopher Hobbs and Steven Foster

BOOKS

Mary Blue
Herbal Foundations: A Guide to Utilizing Medicinal Herbs Effectively

Amanda McQuade Crawford
The Natural Menopause Handbook: Herbs, Nutrition & Other Natural Therapies

Rosalee de la Forêt
Alchemy of Herbs: Transform Everyday Ingredients into Foods and Remedies That Heal

Margi Flint
The Practicing Herbalist: Meeting with Clients, Reading the Body

Lisa Ganora
Herbal Constituents: Foundations of Phytochemistry

Rosemary Gladstar
Herbal Healing for Women

Rosemary Gladstar's Medicinal Herbs: A Beginner's Guide: 33 Healing Herbs to Know, Grow, and Use

Fire Cider!: 101 Zesty Recipes for Health-Boosting Remedies Made with Apple Cider Vinegar

James Green
The Herbal Medicine-Maker's Handbook: A Home Manual

Christopher Hobbs
Christopher Hobbs's Medicinal Mushrooms: The Essential Guide

Medicinal Mushrooms: An Exploration of Tradition, Healing, and Culture (Herbs and Health Series)

David Hoffman
Medical Herbalism: The Science and Practice of Herbal Medicine

Anne McIntyre
The Complete Floral Healer

Deb Soule
Healing Herbs for Women: A Guide to Natural Remedies

How to Move Like a Gardener: Planting and Preparing Medicines from Plants

David Winston
Adaptogens: Herbs for Strength, Stamina, and Stress Relief, 2nd ed., updated and expanded edition

Matthew Wood
The Book of Herbal Wisdom: Using Plants as Medicines

ORGANIZATIONS

American Herbalists Guild (AHG): This organization advocates for access to herbal medicine and high-quality herbal education and supports and promotes clinical herbalism as a profession. Whether you decide to become a member of AHG or not, I highly recommend their list of resources, especially for herbal education. They also put on a yearly symposium that is well worth saving up for.

Herbalists Without Borders: This volunteer-based nonprofit is devoted to providing compassionate holistic care to communities and countries in need and impacted by natural disasters, violent conflicts, poverty, trauma and other access barriers to health and wellness.

Herbalista Health Network: This is an amazing organization to learn about and support! They focus on health care and work to protect health access through clinical services and educational opportunities. They strive for a community-based model of health care that is based on solidarity and not charity. They create community through herbalism by spreading knowledge and keeping costs down through mobile herb clinics. It's truly an inspiring network.

United Plant Savers (UpS): This is an important organization to support. Their mission is to protect and conserve native medicinal plants and their habitat in the United States and Canada. I highly recommend heading over to their site and becoming a member, or at the least go and take a look at the list of endangered and at-risk plants. This way you'll know to avoid buying anything with sandalwood in it, etc.

ONLINE EDUCATION

Chestnut School of Herbal Medicine
https://chestnutherbs.com

David Winston's Center For Herbal Studies
https://herbalstudies.net

Heartstone Center for Earth Essentials
https://heart-stone.com

Mary Blue Herbal Foundations
https://maryblueherbalist.com

Rosemary Gladstar's The Science & Art of Herbalism
https://scienceandartofherbalism.com

Wildflower School of Botanical Medicine
https://wildflowerherbschool.com

ON-SITE EDUCATION

Make sure to also contact your local herb farm or a local herbalist to see if they are offering programs. And, again, check out the AHG website for more great options!

ArborVitae School of Traditional Herbalism

CommonWealth Center for Holistic Herbalism

David Winston's Center for Herbal Studies

Jim McDonald Herbcraft

Mary Blue Herbal Foundations

Northeast School of Botanical Medicine

Old Ways Herbal

Rootwork Herbals

Sacred Vibes: The Art and Practice of Spiritual Herbalism

Vermont Center for Integrative Herbalism

Wildflower School of Botanical Medicine

ONLINE RESOURCES

7song: https://7song.com

Henriette Kress: https://henriettes-herb.com

Jim McDonald: https://herbcraft.org

Nicole Telkes: https://wildflowerherbschool.com and
http://nicoletelkes.com

HERB FARMS

I again would suggest looking for an herb farm local to where you live, but if you don't have access to a local farm here are a few options for ordering herbs online, in addition to our farm Herbal Revolution Farm and Apothecary. Not all farms are certified organic but still practice organic methods; then there are also farms that are conventional and use chemicals. So always make sure you're getting clean, chemical-free, non-GMO herbs.

Healing Spirit Herb Farm

Meeting House Farm

Oshala Herb Farm

Soul Fire Farm

Zack Woods Herb Farm

HERBAL PRODUCT BUSINESSES

Avena Botanicals

Farmacy Herbs

Good Fight Herb Co.

Herbal Revolution

Herbalist & Alchemist, Inc.

Sacred Vibes Apothecary

Sovereignty Herbs

HERB SEED AND PLANT COMPANIES

Fedco Seeds

High Mowing Organic Seeds

Johnny's Selected Seeds

Organic Harvest (herb plug trays)

Strictly Medicinal Seeds

PODCASTS

Herbal Radio

Herbal Action Podcast

Herbal Highway

Medicine Stories

The Holistic Herbalism Podcast

Wild Spirit

INSTAGRAM HERBALISTS I ENJOY FOLLOWING

@empresskarenmrose

@herbalistafreeclinic

@herbalistwithoutborders

@herbcrafter

@laherbalistcollective

@maryblueherbalist

@milkandhoneyherbs

@ofthespirit

@ritual_botanica

@solidarity.apothecary

@thehillbillyafrican

@themedicinegardener

INSTAGRAM HERBAL PRODUCT BUSINESSES

@goodfightherbco

@ravenscrestbotanicals

@redmoonherbs

@ritualbotanicals

@sacredvibesapothecary

@sovereigntyherbs

@tangledrootbotanicals

@wellfedapothecary

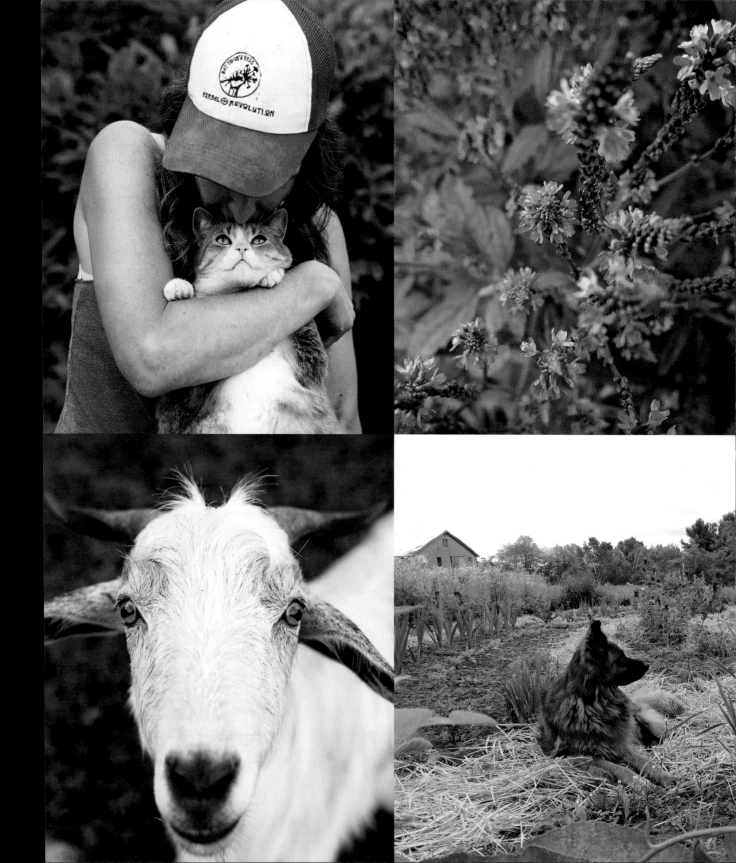

ACKNOWLEDGMENTS

I'd like to take this opportunity to thank my loving and supportive parents, Pat and Ray; my sister, Tara; and my amazing partner, Gustaf.

To all my herbal teachers, mentors and colleagues, thank you for sharing your knowledge—Rosemary Gladstar, Mary Blue, Sheila Kingsbury, Nikki Telkes and David Winston to name just a few.

Big thanks to Page Street Publishing for making this all happen, and to Sarah Monroe, my editor, for all her patience and support during this process. Thanks to Erin Little for all your hard work and gorgeous photographs, and Kristin Dillion for the magic you bring to each photo shoot; the cover is stunning.

Big love to all the amazing herbalists out there who are on the ground supporting communities, educating others and spreading knowledge of the plants.

And of course, my deep gratitude to the plants. Without them, this book wouldn't exist.

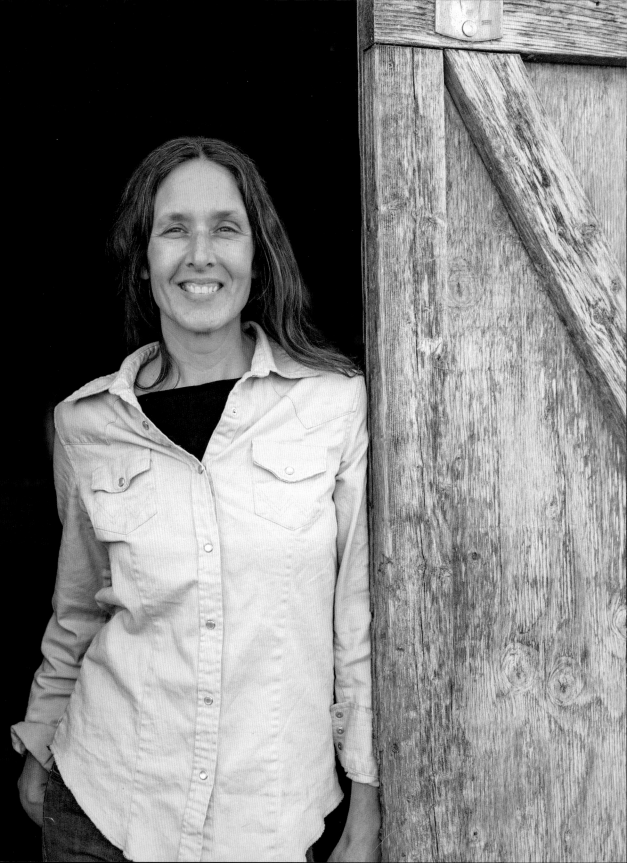

ABOUT THE AUTHOR

Katheryn Langelier (Kathi) is the founder, farmer and formulator for Herbal Revolution Farm and Apothecary, located in Union, Maine. She has received numerous awards over the years for her formulas from organizations such as the American Herbalists Guild, International Herb Symposium and New England Made Shows. In 2019, she received an award for being the Best Home-Based Business for Maine and all of New England from the Small Business Administration. Kathi has been featured in the *Boston Globe, New York Times, Mother Earth News, Maine Women Magazine, Bangor Daily News, Penobscot Bay Pilot* and *HerbalGram* for her work with the Fire Cider 3 and Tradition Not Trademark. Her products have been featured in *Down East Magazine, New England Made Shows* and the *New York Post.*

Kathi currently oversees 5 acres (2 ha) of medicinal herb production on her certified organic farm. All the herbs and vegetables grown on the farm are used to create Herbal Revolution's delicious, effective and versatile herbal products. Herbal Revolution offers an extensive line of elixirs, tinctures, teas, vinegar tonics, flower essences and body products.

There are some exciting projects Kathi is working on, including creating gardens and trails at the Herbal Revolution production location (headquarters), located 2 miles (3.2 km) down the road from the farm. She has big plans of opening a café and retail space and also creating a space for herbal programs, workshops, community outreach and clinical work.

She studied clinical herbalism with David Winston, Leslie Alexander and Leslita Williams, and has spent the last twenty-five years of her life following her passion for organic farming, herbal medicine and community wellness with great dedication. When Kathi's not working on the farm or at headquarters, she loves hiking, swimming, playing with her cashmere goats, eating delicious food, traveling and having new experiences, laughing her ass off and spending time with her family and partner, Gus.

To learn more, visit www.herbalrev.com and follow her on social media.

INDEX